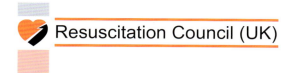

Resuscitation Council (UK)

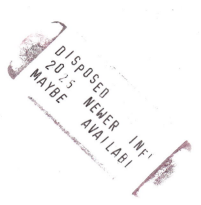
Resus

2005

Decemb

Edited by Anthony J. Handley

Published by the Resuscitation Council (UK)
5th Floor, Tavistock House North
Tavistock Square
London WC1H 9HR

Tel: 020 7388 4678   • Fax: 020 7383 0773   • E-mail: enquiries@resus.org.uk
• Website: www.resus.org.uk
Registered charity no. 286360

ISBN 1-903812-10-0

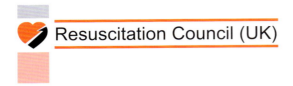

Foreword

The Resuscitation Council (UK) is a registered charity formed in August 1981 by a group of medical practitioners from a variety of specialities who shared an interest in resuscitation. The objectives of the Council are:

- To produce guidelines for resuscitation procedures.
- To publish national standards for resuscitation and provide guidance on how they can be achieved.
- To promote the teaching of resuscitation in accordance with the established guidelines.
- To study and improve resuscitation teaching techniques.
- To encourage and fund research in resuscitation.
- To foster good working relations between all organisations involved in resuscitation.
- To design and publish training materials for high-quality resuscitation courses.
- To provide administrative support for resuscitation training courses.

Several members of the Executive Committee of the RC (UK) contribute to the activities of the European Resuscitation Council and International Liaison Committee on Resuscitation (ILCOR); these bodies are responsible for training, research, and guideline setting worldwide.

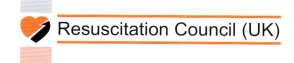 Resuscitation Council (UK)

Contents

Throughout this publication the masculine is used to denote the masculine or feminine.

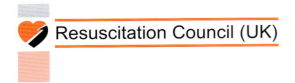
Resuscitation Council (UK)

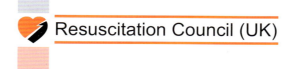Resuscitation Council (UK)

Introduction

Dr. Michael Colquhoun
Chairman Resuscitation Council (UK)

Dr. Jerry Nolan
Vice-chairman Resuscitation Council (UK)
Co-chairman International Liaison Committee on Resuscitation (ILCOR)

The simultaneous publication of Guidelines 2000 for Cardiopulmonary Resuscitation and Emergency Cardiovascular Care in both Resuscitation[1] and Circulation[2] provided the basis for the first international resuscitation guidelines, and represented a milestone in international collaboration to improve the practice and teaching of resuscitation medicine. Representatives from the world's major resuscitation organisations reached this consensus only after exhaustive review of the published literature and extensive debate at consensus meetings. The review process was thorough and provided the best evidence-based approach to the resuscitation of patients of all ages. The guidelines that arose from this process were adopted internationally with only minor modifications required by local custom, practice, or availability of drugs.

This review process was repeated during 2004/5. It was led by the International Liaison Committee on Resuscitation (ILCOR) and culminated in the 2005 International Consensus Conference on Emergency Cardiovascular Care (ECC) and Cardiopulmonary Resuscitation (CPR) Science with Treatment Recommendations, hosted by the American Heart Association (AHA). The summary science statements and treatment recommendations from this conference have been published: *2005 International Consensus on Cardiopulmonary Resuscitation and Emergency Cardiovascular Care Science with Treatment Recommendations* (CoSTR).[3] This document formed the scientific basis for the European Resuscitation Council (ERC) Guidelines for Resuscitation 2005.[4] The Resuscitation Council (UK) Guidelines 2005 in this document are an abbreviated version of the ERC guidelines and differ from other international organisations only in minor ways.

These latest guidelines contain some treatment recommendations and changes in practice based on new scientific evidence that has accrued since 2000. Consistency in practice among countries provides the basis for the large trials necessary to establish best practice, and the further development of such international collaboration is greatly to be encouraged. Similarly, consistent collection and reporting of audit data in registries that enable comparison between systems does much to improve practice and ensure that the victims of sudden cardiac arrest are given the best chance of successful resuscitation. These current guidelines reflect improvements in practice resulting from research and audit, encouraged by the co-operation that exists within the international resuscitation community.

Resuscitation Council (UK)

The adult basic and advanced algorithms and paediatric resuscitation algorithms have been updated to reflect changes in the guidelines. Every effort has been made to keep these algorithms simple, yet make them applicable to cardiac arrest victims in most circumstances. Rescuers begin CPR if the victim is unconscious or unresponsive and not breathing normally (ignoring occasional gasps). A single compression-ventilation (CV) ratio of 30:2 is used by the single rescuer of an adult or child (excluding neonate) out of hospital, and for all adult CPR. This single ratio is designed to simplify teaching, promote skill retention, increase the number of compressions given, and decrease interruption to compressions. Once a defibrillator is attached, if a shockable rhythm is confirmed, a single shock is delivered. Irrespective of the resultant rhythm, chest compressions and ventilations (two minutes with a CV ratio of 30:2) are resumed immediately after the shock to minimise the 'no-flow' time.

Recent evidence indicates that unnecessary interruptions to chest compressions occur frequently both in and out of hospital.[5-7] Resuscitation instructors must emphasise the importance of minimising interruptions to chest compression.

Several of the treatment recommendations in these guidelines represent significant changes in the way resuscitation is delivered. It will take time for courses and training materials to be updated and for this change in practice to be disseminated to healthcare professionals and laypeople by resuscitation trainers. As this transition is made there will inevitably be some variation in practice between individuals and healthcare organisations. The updated guidelines in Guidelines 2005 do not define the only way that resuscitation should be achieved, they merely represent a widely accepted view of how resuscitation can be undertaken both safely and effectively. The publication of new treatment recommendations does not imply that current clinical care is either unsafe or ineffective.

The process leading to the publication of the guidelines has entailed considerable work by many individuals over a protracted period. The Resuscitation Council (UK) would like to thank all the individuals and organisations that have contributed to the process and made this publication possible.

References

1. American Heart Association in collaboration with International Liaison Committee on Resuscitation. Guidelines for Cardiopulmonary Resuscitation and Emergency Cardiovascular Care---An International Consensus on Science. Resuscitation 2000;46:3-430.

2. American Heart Association in collaboration with International Liaison Committee on Resuscitation. Guidelines 2000 for Cardiopulmonary Resuscitation and Emergency Cardiovascular Care. Circulation 2000;102(suppl):I1-I384.

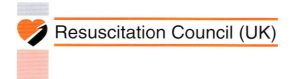

Resuscitation Council (UK)

3. International Liaison Committee on Resuscitation. 2005 International Consensus on Cardiopulmonary Resuscitation and Emergency Cardiovascular Care Science with Treatment Recommendations. Resuscitation 2005;67:157-341.

4. European Resuscitation Council. European Resuscitation Council Guidelines for Resuscitation 2005. Resuscitation 2005;67(Suppl. 1):S1-S190.

5. Wik L, Kramer-Johansen J, Myklebust H, et al. Quality of cardiopulmonary resuscitation during out-of-hospital cardiac arrest. JAMA 2005;293:299-304.

6. Abella BS, Alvarado JP, Myklebust H, et al. Quality of cardiopulmonary resuscitation during in-hospital cardiac arrest. JAMA 2005;293:305-10.

7. Abella BS, Sandbo N, Vassilatos P, et al. Chest compression rates during cardiopulmonary resuscitation are suboptimal: a prospective study during in-hospital cardiac arrest. Circulation 2005;111:428-34.

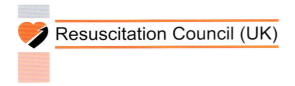

Resuscitation Council (UK)

Adult Basic Life Support

Introduction

This section contains the guidelines for out-of-hospital, single rescuer, adult basic life support (BLS). Like the other guidelines in this publication, it is based on the document *2005 International Consensus on Cardiopulmonary Resuscitation and Emergency Cardiovascular Care Science with Treatment Recommendations* (CoSTR), which was published in November 2005. Basic life support implies that no equipment is employed other than a protective device.

Guideline changes

There are two main underlying themes in the BLS section of CoSTR: the need to increase the number of chest compressions given to a victim of cardiac arrest, and the importance of simplifying guidelines to aid acquisition and retention of BLS skills, particularly for laypersons.

It is well documented that interruptions in chest compression are common[1] and are associated with a reduced chance of survival for the victim.[2] The 'perfect' solution is to deliver continuous compressions whilst giving ventilations independently. This is possible when the victim has an advanced airway in place, and is discussed in the adult advanced life support (ALS) section. Chest-compression-only CPR is another way to increase the number of compressions given and will, by definition, eliminate pauses. It is effective for a limited period only (about 5 min) [3] and is not recommended as standard management of out-of-hospital cardiac arrest.

The following changes in the BLS guidelines have been made to reflect the greater importance placed on chest compression, and to attempt to reduce the number and duration of pauses:

1) Make a diagnosis of cardiac arrest if a victim is unresponsive and not breathing normally.

2) Teach rescuers to place their hands in the centre of the chest, rather than to spend more time using the 'rib margin' method.

3) Give each rescue breath over 1 sec rather than 2 sec.

4) Use a ratio of compressions to ventilations of 30:2 for all adult victims of sudden cardiac arrest. Use this same ratio for children when attended by a lay rescuer.

5) For an adult victim, omit the initial 2 rescue breaths and give 30 compressions immediately after cardiac arrest is established.

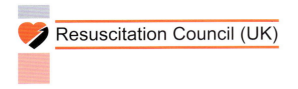 Resuscitation Council (UK)

Adult Basic Life Support

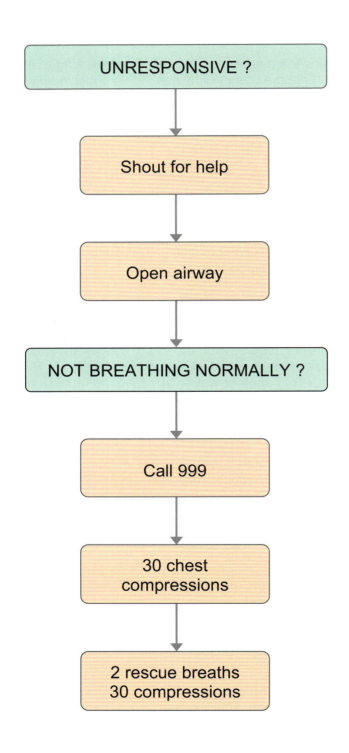

UNRESPONSIVE ?

↓

Shout for help

↓

Open airway

↓

NOT BREATHING NORMALLY ?

↓

Call 999

↓

30 chest compressions

↓

2 rescue breaths
30 compressions

To aid teaching and learning, the sequence of actions has been simplified. In some cases, simplification has been based on recently published evidence; in others there was no evidence that the previous, more complicated, sequence had any beneficial effect on survival.

There are other changes in the guidelines. In particular, allowance has been made for the rescuer who is unable or unwilling to perform rescue breathing. It is well recorded that reluctance to perform mouth-to-mouth ventilation, in spite of the lack of evidence of risk, inhibits many would-be rescuers from attempting any form of resuscitation. These guidelines encourage chest compression alone in such circumstances.

Guidelines 2000 introduced the concept of checking for 'signs of a circulation'. This change was made because of the evidence that relying on a check of the carotid pulse to diagnose cardiac arrest is unreliable and time-consuming, mainly, but not exclusively, when attempted by non-healthcare professionals.[4] Subsequent studies have shown that checking for breathing is also prone to error, particularly as agonal gasps are frequently misdiagnosed as normal breathing.[5] In Guidelines 2005 the absence of breathing, in a non-responsive victim, continues to be the main sign of cardiac arrest. Also highlighted is the need to identify agonal gasps as another, positive, indication to start CPR.

Finally, there is recognition that delivering chest compressions is tiring. It is now recommended that, where more than one rescuer is present, another should take over the compressions (with a minimum of delay) about every 2 min to prevent fatigue and maintain the quality of performance.

Adult BLS sequence

Basic life support consists of the following sequence of actions:

1   **Make sure the victim, any bystanders, and you are safe.**

2   **Check the victim for a response.**
- Gently shake his shoulders and ask loudly, 'Are you all right?'

3 A   **If he responds:**
- Leave him in the position in which you find him provided there is no further danger.
- Try to find out what is wrong with him and get help if needed.
- Reassess him regularly.

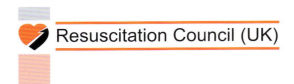
Resuscitation Council (UK)

3 B **If he does <u>not</u> respond**:
- Shout for help.
- Turn the victim onto his back and then open the airway using head tilt and chin lift:
  - Place your hand on his forehead and gently tilt his head back.
  - With your fingertips under the point of the victim's chin, lift the chin to open the airway.

4 **Keeping the airway open, look, listen, and feel for normal breathing.**
- Look for chest movement.
- Listen at the victim's mouth for breath sounds.
- Feel for air on your cheek.

In the first few minutes after cardiac arrest, a victim may be barely breathing, or taking infrequent, noisy, gasps. Do not confuse this with normal breathing.

Look, listen, and feel for **no more** than **10 sec** to determine if the victim is breathing normally. If you have any doubt whether breathing is normal, act as if it is **not** normal.

5 A **If he <u>is</u> breathing normally:**
- Turn him into the recovery position (**see below**).
- Send or go for help, or call for an ambulance.
- Check for continued breathing.

5 B **If he is <u>not</u> breathing normally:**
- Ask someone to call for an ambulance or, if you are on your own, do this yourself; you may need to leave the victim. Start chest compression as follows:
  - Kneel by the side of the victim.
  - Place the heel of one hand in the centre of the victim's chest.
  - Place the heel of your other hand on top of the first hand.
  - Interlock the fingers of your hands and ensure that pressure is not applied over the victim's ribs. Do not apply any pressure over the upper abdomen or the bottom end of the bony sternum (breastbone).
  - Position yourself vertically above the victim's chest and, with your arms straight, press down on the sternum 4 - 5 cm.
  - After each compression, release all the pressure on the chest without losing contact between your hands and the sternum. Repeat at a rate of about 100 times a minute (a little less than 2 compressions a second).
  - Compression and release should take an equal amount of time.

6 A Combine chest compression with rescue breaths.

- After 30 compressions open the airway again using head tilt and chin lift.

- Pinch the soft part of the victim's nose closed, using the index finger and thumb of your hand on his forehead.

- Allow his mouth to open, but maintain chin lift.

- Take a normal breath and place your lips around his mouth, making sure that you have a good seal.

- Blow steadily into his mouth whilst watching for his chest to rise; take about one second to make his chest rise as in normal breathing; this is an effective rescue breath.

- Maintaining head tilt and chin lift, take your mouth away from the victim and watch for his chest to fall as air comes out.

- Take another normal breath and blow into the victim's mouth once more to give a total of two effective rescue breaths. Then return your hands without delay to the correct position on the sternum and give a further 30 chest compressions.

- Continue with chest compressions and rescue breaths in a ratio of 30:2.

- Stop to recheck the victim only if he starts breathing **normally**; otherwise **do not interrupt resuscitation.**

If your rescue breaths do not make the chest rise as in normal breathing, then before your next attempt:

- Check the victim's mouth and remove any visible obstruction.

- Recheck that there is adequate head tilt and chin lift.

- Do not attempt more than two breaths each time before returning to chest compressions.

If there is more than one rescuer present, another should take over CPR about every 2 min to prevent fatigue. Ensure the minimum of delay during the changeover of rescuers.

6 B Chest-compression-only CPR.

- If you are not able, or are unwilling, to give rescue breaths, give chest compressions only.

- If chest compressions only are given, these should be continuous at a rate of 100 a minute.

- Stop to recheck the victim only if he starts breathing **normally**; otherwise do not interrupt resuscitation.

7 Continue resuscitation until:

- qualified help arrives and takes over,

- the victim starts breathing normally, or

- you become exhausted.

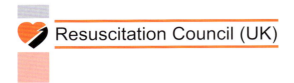

Resuscitation Council (UK)

Explanatory notes

Risk to the rescuer

The safety of both the rescuer and victim are paramount during a resuscitation attempt. There have been few incidents of rescuers suffering adverse effects from undertaking CPR, with only isolated reports of infections such as tuberculosis (TB) and severe acute respiratory distress syndrome (SARS). Transmission of HIV during CPR has never been reported. There have been no human studies to address the effectiveness of barrier devices during CPR; however, laboratory studies have shown that certain filters, or barrier devices with one-way valves, prevent oral bacteria transmission from the victim to the rescuer during mouth-to-mouth ventilation. Rescuers should take appropriate safety precautions where feasible, especially if the victim is known to have a serious infection, such as TB.

Initial rescue breaths

During the first few minutes after non-asphyxial cardiac arrest the blood oxygen content remains high. Ventilation is, therefore, less important than chest compression at this time.

It is well recognised that skill acquisition and retention are aided by simplification of the BLS sequence of actions. It is also recognised that rescuers are frequently unwilling to carry out mouth-to-mouth ventilation for a variety of reasons, including fear of infection and distaste for the procedure. For these reasons, and to emphasise the priority of chest compressions, it is recommended that, in most adults, CPR should start with chest compressions rather than initial ventilations.

Jaw thrust

The jaw thrust technique is not recommended for lay rescuers because it is difficult to learn and perform. Therefore, the lay rescuer should open the airway using a head-tilt-chin-lift manoeuvre.

Agonal gasps

Agonal gasps are present in up to 40% of cardiac arrest victims. Laypeople should, therefore, be taught to begin CPR if the victim is unconscious (unresponsive) and not breathing normally. It should be emphasised during training that agonal gasps occur commonly in the first few minutes after sudden cardiac arrest. They are an indication for starting CPR immediately and should not be confused with normal breathing.

Mouth-to-nose ventilation

Mouth-to-nose ventilation is an effective alternative to mouth-to-mouth ventilation. It may be considered if the victim's mouth is seriously injured or cannot be opened, the rescuer is assisting a victim in the water, or a mouth-to-mouth seal is difficult to achieve.

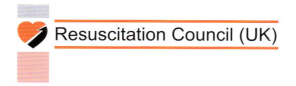

Resuscitation Council (UK)

Mouth-to-tracheostomy ventilation

Mouth-to-tracheostomy ventilation may be used for a victim with a tracheostomy tube or tracheal stoma who requires rescue breathing.

Bag-mask ventilation

Considerable practice and skill are required to use a bag and mask for ventilation. The lone rescuer has to be able to open the airway with a jaw thrust whilst simultaneously holding the mask to the victim's face. It is a technique that is appropriate only for lay rescuers who work in highly specialised areas, such as where there is a risk of cyanide poisoning or exposure to other toxic agents. There are other specific circumstances in which non-healthcare providers receive extended training in first aid which could include training, and retraining, in the use of bag-mask ventilation. The same strict training that applies to healthcare professionals should be followed and the two-person technique is preferable.

Chest compression

In most circumstances it will be possible to identify the correct hand position for chest compression without removing the victim's clothes. If in any doubt, remove outer clothing.

In Guidelines 2000 a method was recommended for finding the correct hand position by placing one finger on the lower end of the sternum and sliding the other hand down to it. It has been shown that the same hand position can be found more quickly if rescuers are taught to 'place the heel of your hand in the centre of the chest with the other hand on top', provided the teaching includes a demonstration of placing the hands in the middle of the lower half of the sternum.[6]

Whilst performing chest compression:

    a) Each time compressions are resumed, the rescuer should place his hands without delay 'in the centre of the chest'.

    b) Compress the chest at a rate of about 100 a minute.

    c) Pay attention to achieving the full compression depth of 4-5 cm (for an adult).

    d) Allow the chest to recoil completely after each compression.

    e) Take approximately the same amount of time for compression and relaxation.

    f) Minimise interruptions in chest compression.

    g) Do not rely on a palpable carotid or femoral pulse as a gauge of effective arterial flow.

    h) 'Compression rate' refers to the speed at which compressions are given, not the total number delivered in each minute. The number delivered is determined not only by the rate, but also by the number of interruptions to open the airway, deliver rescue breaths, and allow AED analysis.

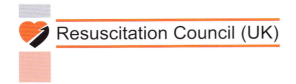

Compression-only CPR

Studies have shown that chest-compression-only CPR may be as effective as combined ventilation and compression in the first few minutes after non-asphyxial arrest. Laypeople should, therefore, be encouraged to do compression-only CPR if they are unable or unwilling to provide rescue breaths, although combined chest compression and ventilation is the better method of CPR.

Over-the-head CPR

Over-the-head CPR for a single rescuer and straddle CPR for two rescuers may be considered for resuscitation in confined spaces.

Recovery position

There are several variations of the recovery position, each with its own advantages. No single position is perfect for all victims. The position should be stable, near a true lateral position with the head dependent, and with no pressure on the chest to impair breathing.

The Resuscitation Council (UK) recommends this sequence of actions to place a victim in the recovery position:

- Remove the victim's spectacles.
- Kneel beside the victim and make sure that both his legs are straight.
- Place the arm nearest to you out at right angles to his body, elbow bent with the hand palm uppermost.
- Bring the far arm across the chest, and hold the back of the hand against the victim's cheek nearest to you.
- With your other hand, grasp the far leg just above the knee and pull it up, keeping the foot on the ground.
- Keeping his hand pressed against his cheek, pull on the far leg to roll the victim towards you onto his side.
- Adjust the upper leg so that both the hip and knee are bent at right angles.
- Tilt the head back to make sure the airway remains open.
- Adjust the hand under the cheek, if necessary, to keep the head tilted.
- Check breathing regularly.

If the victim has to be kept in the recovery position for **more than 30 min** turn him to the opposite side to relieve the pressure on the lower arm.

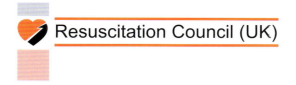

Choking

Recognition

Because recognition of choking (airway obstruction by a foreign body) is the key to successful outcome, it is important not to confuse this emergency with fainting, heart attack, seizure, or other conditions that may cause sudden respiratory distress, cyanosis, or loss of consciousness.

Foreign bodies may cause either mild or severe airway obstruction. The signs and symptoms enabling differentiation between mild and severe airway obstruction are summarised in the table below. It is important to ask the conscious victim 'Are you choking?'

General signs of choking	
<ul><li>Attack occurs while eating</li><li>Victim may clutch his neck</li></ul>	
Signs of mild airway obstruction	**Signs of severe airway obstruction**
Response to question 'Are you choking?' <ul><li>Victim speaks and answers yes</li></ul> *Other signs* <ul><li>Victim is able to speak, cough, and breathe</li></ul>	*Response to question 'Are you choking?'* <ul><li>Victim unable to speak</li><li>Victim may respond by nodding</li></ul> *Other signs* <ul><li>Victim unable to breathe</li><li>Breathing sounds wheezy</li><li>Attempts at coughing are silent</li><li>Victim may be unconscious</li></ul>

Adult choking sequence

(This sequence is also suitable for use in children over the age of 1 year)

1   **If the victim shows signs of mild airway obstruction:**
   - Encourage him to continue coughing, but do nothing else.

2   **If the victim shows signs of severe airway obstruction and is conscious:**
   - Give up to five back blows.
     - o Stand to the side and slightly behind the victim.
     - o Support the chest with one hand and lean the victim well forwards so that when the obstructing object is dislodged it comes out of the mouth rather than goes further down the airway.
     - o Give **up to** five sharp blows between the shoulder blades with the heel of your other hand.

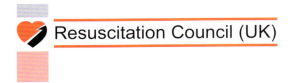
Resuscitation Council (UK)

Adult choking treatment

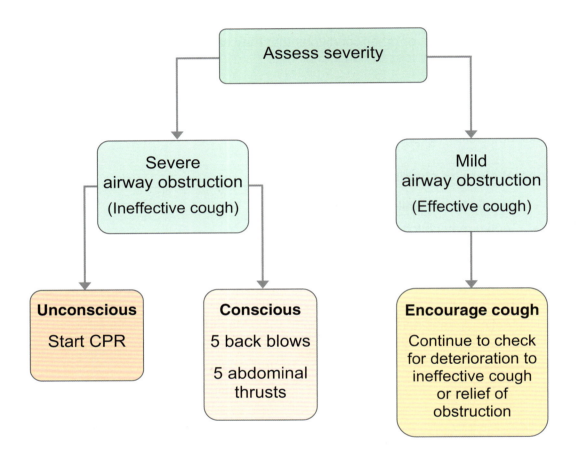

- Check to see if each back blow has relieved the airway obstruction. The aim is to relieve the obstruction with each blow rather than necessarily to give all five.

- If five back blows fail to relieve the airway obstruction give up to five abdominal thrusts.
  - Stand behind the victim and put both arms round the upper part of his abdomen.
  - Lean the victim forwards.
  - Clench your fist and place it between the umbilicus (navel) and the bottom end of the sternum (breastbone).
  - Grasp this hand with your other hand and pull sharply inwards and upwards.
  - Repeat up to five times.

- If the obstruction is still not relieved, continue alternating five back blows with five abdominal thrusts.

3   If the victim becomes unconscious:

- Support the victim carefully to the ground.

- Immediately call an ambulance.

- Begin CPR (from 5B of the Adult BLS Sequence). Healthcare providers, trained and experienced in feeling for a carotid pulse, should initiate chest compressions even if a pulse is present in the unconscious choking victim.

Explanatory notes

Following successful treatment for choking, foreign material may nevertheless remain in the upper or lower respiratory tract and cause complications later. Victims with a persistent cough, difficulty swallowing, or with the sensation of an object being still stuck in the throat should therefore be referred for a medical opinion.

Abdominal thrusts can cause serious internal injuries and all victims receiving abdominal thrusts should be examined for injury by a doctor.

Resuscitation of children and victims of drowning

Both ventilation and compression are important for victims of cardiac arrest when the oxygen stores become depleted – about 4-6 min after collapse from ventricular fibrillation (VF), and immediately after collapse for victims of asphyxial arrest. Previous guidelines tried to take into account the difference in causation, and recommended that victims of identifiable asphyxia (drowning; trauma; intoxication) and children should receive 1 min of CPR before the lone rescuer left the victim to get help. The majority of cases of sudden cardiac arrest out of hospital, however, occur in adults and are of cardiac origin due to VF. These additional recommendations, therefore, added to the complexity of the guidelines whilst affecting only a minority of victims.

Also important is that many children do not receive resuscitation because potential rescuers fear causing harm. This fear is unfounded; it is far better to use the adult BLS sequence for resuscitation of a child than to do nothing.

For ease of teaching and retention, therefore, laypeople should be taught that the adult sequence may also be used for children who are not responsive and not breathing.

The following minor modifications to the adult sequence will, however, make it even more suitable for use in children:

- Give five initial rescue breaths before starting chest compressions (adult sequence of actions 5B).
- If you are on your own perform CPR for approximately 1 min before going for help.
- Compress the chest by approximately one-third of its depth. Use two fingers for an infant under 1 year; use one or two hands for a child over 1 year as needed to achieve an adequate depth of compression.

The same modifications of five initial breaths, and 1 min of CPR by the lone rescuer before getting help, may improve outcome for victims of drowning. This modification should be taught only to those who have a specific duty of care to potential drowning victims (e.g. lifeguards).

Drowning is easily identified. It can be difficult, on the other hand, for a layperson to determine whether cardiorespiratory arrest has been caused by trauma or intoxication. These victims should, therefore, be managed according to the standard protocol.

References

1   Van Alem A, B Sanou, R Koster. Interruption of CPR with the use of the AED in out of hospital cardiac arrest. Med. Ann Emerg Med 2003;42:449-57.

2   Eftestol T, Sunde K, Steen PA. Effects of interrupting precordial compressions on the calculated probability of defibrillation success during out-of-hospital cardiac arrest. Circulation 2002;105:2270-3.

3   Hallstrom A, Cobb L, Johnson E, Copass M. Cardiopulmonary resuscitation by chest compression alone or with mouth-to-mouth ventilation. N Engl J Med 2000;342:1546-1553.

4   Bahr J, Klingler H, Panzer W, Rode H, Kettler D. Skills of lay people in checking the carotid pulse. Resuscitation 1997;35:23-26.

5   Hauff SR, Rea TD, Culley LL, Kerry F, Becker L, Eisenberg MS. Factors impeding dispatcher-assisted telephone cardiopulmonary resuscitation. Ann Emerg Med 2003;42:731-7.

6   Handley AJ. Teaching hand placement for chest compression - a simpler technique. Resuscitation 2002; 53:29-36.

Resuscitation Council (UK)

The use of Automated External Defibrillators

Introduction

This section contains guidelines for the use of automated external defibrillators (AEDs) by laypeople, first responders, and healthcare professionals responding with an AED out of hospital. These guidelines are appropriate for all AEDs, including those that are fully automatic. Guidelines for in-hospital use of manual defibrillators are in the adult advanced life support (ALS) section.

Sudden cardiac arrest is a leading cause of death in Europe, affecting about 700,000 individuals a year.[1] Many victims of sudden cardiac arrest can survive if bystanders act immediately while ventricular fibrillation (VF) is still present; successful resuscitation is unlikely once the rhythm has deteriorated to asystole.[2]

Electrical defibrillation is well established as the only effective therapy for cardiac arrest caused by VF or pulseless ventricular tachycardia (VT). The scientific evidence to support early defibrillation is overwhelming; the delay from collapse to delivery of the first shock is the single most important determinant of survival. The chances of successful defibrillation decline at a rate of 7-10% with each minute of delay; basic life support will help to maintain a shockable rhythm but is not a definitive treatment.

The Resuscitation Council (UK) strongly recommends a policy of early attempted defibrillation.

Guideline changes

Although Guidelines 2005 contain recommendations for changes in the sequence of shock delivery, there are no fundamental changes to the sequence of actions, since users should be taught to determine the need for an AED, switch on the machine, attach the electrodes, and follow the prompts.

The main guideline changes are:

1) Place the axillary electrode pad vertically to improve efficiency.

2) If possible, continue CPR whilst the pads are being applied.

3) Program AEDs to deliver a single shock followed by a pause of 2 min for the immediate resumption of CPR (see adult ALS section).

AED Algorithm

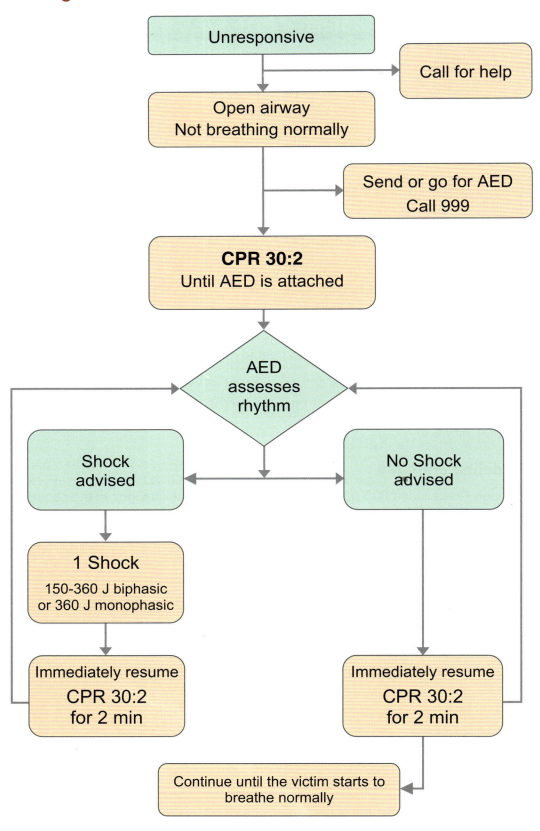

Types of AEDs

AEDs are sophisticated, reliable, safe, computerised devices that deliver defibrillatory shocks to victims of cardiac arrest. They use voice and visual prompts to guide rescuers, and are suitable for use by lay rescuers and healthcare professionals. There are two types of AED: most are semi-automatic, but a few fully-automatic AEDs are available. All AEDs analyse the victim's rhythm, determine the need for a shock, and then deliver a shock. A semi-automatic AED advises the need for a shock, but this has to be delivered by the operator when prompted. Some semi-automatic AEDs have the facility to enable the operator (normally a healthcare professional) to override the device and deliver a shock manually, independently of any prompts.

Sequence of actions when using an AED

The following sequence is for the use of both semi-automatic and automatic AEDs.

1   **Make sure the victim, any bystanders, and you are safe.**
    - If two rescuers are present, assign tasks.

2   **If the victim is unresponsive and not breathing normally:**
    - Send someone for the AED and to call for an ambulance. If you are on your own do this yourself; you may need to leave the victim.

3   **Start CPR according to the guidelines for BLS.**

4   **As soon as the AED arrives:**
    - Switch on the AED and attach the electrode pads. If more than one rescuer is present, continue CPR whilst this is done. (Some AEDs may automatically switch on when the AED lid is opened).
    - Follow the voice / visual prompts.
    - Ensure that nobody touches the victim whilst the AED is analysing the rhythm.

5 A   **If a shock <u>is</u> indicated:**
    - Ensure that nobody touches the victim.
    - Push the shock button as directed.
      (Fully-automatic AEDs will deliver the shock automatically).
    - Continue as directed by the voice / visual prompts.

5 B   **If <u>no</u> shock is indicated:**
    - Immediately resume CPR using a ratio of 30 compressions to 2 rescue breaths.
    - Continue as directed by the voice / visual prompts.

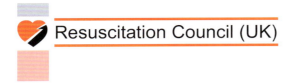
Resuscitation Council (UK)

6   **Continue to follow the AED prompts until:**
   - qualified help arrives and takes over,
   - the victim starts to breathe normally, or
   - you become exhausted.

Placement of AED pads

The victim's chest must be sufficiently exposed to enable correct electrode pad placement. Chest hair will prevent the pads adhering to the skin and will interfere with electrical contact. Shave the chest only if the hair is excessive, and even then spend as little time as possible on this. Do not delay defibrillation if a razor is not immediately available.

Place one AED pad to the right of the sternum, below the clavicle. Place the other pad in the mid-axillary line, approximately level with the V6 ECG electrode position or the female breast. This position should be clear of any breast tissue. It is important that this electrode is placed sufficiently laterally. In order to improve efficiency, place the mid-axillary pad with its long axis vertical.[3]

Although most AED pads are labelled left and right, or carry a picture of their correct placement, it does not matter if they are reversed. It is important to teach that if an 'error' is made, the pads should not be removed and replaced as this wastes time and they may well not adhere adequately when re-attached.

CPR before defibrillation

Immediate defibrillation, as soon as an AED becomes available, has always been a key element in guidelines and teaching. This concept has recently been challenged. There are studies showing that when the time between calling for an ambulance and its arrival exceeds 5 min, a period of chest compression before defibrillation may improve survival. However, in these studies CPR was performed by paramedics, who also protected the airway by intubation and delivered 100% oxygen. Similar results may not be achievable by lay responders. For this reason Guidelines 2005 continues to recommend an immediate shock as soon as the AED is available.

Voice prompts

Voice prompts are usually programmable and it is recommended that they be set as follows:
   - a single shock only when a shockable rhythm is detected;
   - no rhythm, breathing, or pulse check after the shock;
   - a voice prompt for immediate resumption of CPR after the shock;
   - two min allowed for CPR before a voice prompt to assess the rhythm, breathing, or a pulse is given.

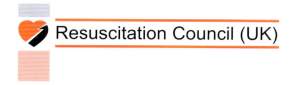
Resuscitation Council (UK)

AED use by healthcare professionals

All healthcare professionals should consider the use of an AED to be an integral component of basic life support. Early defibrillation should be available throughout all hospitals, outpatient medical facilities, and clinics. An adequate number of staff should be trained to enable a first shock to be provided within 3 min of collapse anywhere in the hospital. Hospitals should monitor collapse-to-first-shock intervals and monitor resuscitation outcomes.

AED use by trained lay first responders

AEDs should be deployed within a medically-controlled system under the direction of a medical adviser. This may be a doctor from any medical discipline who has clinical expertise in resuscitation. Medical advisers should be career-grade doctors including consultants, GP principals, and other equivalents in the Voluntary Aid Societies, commercial and charitable organisations, and the Defence Medical Services. The 'medical director/adviser' is responsible for ensuring that controls are in place to ensure adequate training of AED users, with periodic refresher training. This training and retraining must be provided by appropriately qualified individuals, for example resuscitation training officers, community defibrillation officers, medical or nursing staff, ambulance service trainers, and other individuals such as first aid trainers accredited in AED training. Basic life support skills must also be taught, assessed, and refreshed in accordance with current guidelines.

Children

Smaller, paediatric, self-adhesive pads, that attenuate the delivered current during defibrillation, are available for use with AEDs. Standard AEDs are suitable for use in children older than 8 years. In children between 1 and 8 years paediatric pads or a paediatric mode should be used if available; if not, the AED should be used as it is. There is insufficient evidence to support a recommendation for or against the use of AEDs in children less than 1 year.

Public access defibrillation (PAD)

Public access defibrillation (PAD) and first-responder programmes are now widespread. An important factor contributing to the high success rates of PAD is the short response time from collapse to resuscitation.[4] Some ambulance trusts have reduced the time to defibrillation by using trained, lay, responders. Although such a strategy has been reported to improve the incidence of return of spontaneous circulation and survival to hospital admission, there is as yet limited evidence of increased survival to hospital discharge.[5] To have the greatest impact, such schemes should be introduced where the risk of cardiac arrest is highest. It has been suggested that for public access schemes to be cost-effective, the probability of cardiac arrest occurring in the location should be at least once every two years.[6]

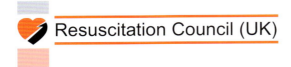

Resuscitation Council (UK)

References

1. Sans S, Kesteloot H, Kromhout D. The burden of cardiovascular diseases mortality in Europe. Task Force of the European Society of Cardiology on Cardiovascular Mortality and Morbidity Statistics in Europe. Eur Heart J 1997;18:1231-48.

2. Larsen MP, Eisenberg MS, Cummins RO, Hallstrom AP. Predicting survival from out-of-hospital cardiac arrest: a graphic model. Ann Emerg Med 1993;22:1652-8.

3. Deakin CD, Sado DM, Petley GW, Clewlow F. Is the orientation of the apical defibrillation paddle of importance during manual external defibrillation? Resuscitation 2003;56:15-8.

4. Whitfield R, Colquhoun M, Newcombe R, Davies C. S, Boyle R. The Department of Health National Defibrillator Programme: analysis of downloads from 250 deployments of public access defibrillators. Resuscitation 2005;64:269 – 77.

5. Van Alem AP, Vrenken RH, de Vos R, Tijssen JG, Koster RW. Use of automated external defibrillator by first responders in out of hospital cardiac arrest: prospective controlled trial. BMJ 2003;327:1312.

6. Becker DE. Assessment and management of cardiovascular urgencies and emergencies: cognitive and technical considerations. Anaesthesia Progress 1988;35:212-7.

Prevention of in-hospital cardiac arrest and decisions about cardiopulmonary resuscitation

Introduction

This new section of the Resuscitation Council (UK) guidelines stresses the importance of preventing cardiac arrest in all age groups, and of identifying patients for whom cardiopulmonary resuscitation is inappropriate.

Prevention of in-hospital cardiac arrest

Rates of survival and complete physiological recovery following in-hospital cardiac arrest are poor in all age groups. For example, fewer than 20% of adult patients having an in-hospital cardiac arrest will survive to go home.[1] Cardiac arrest is rare in both pregnant women and children, but outcomes after in-hospital arrest are also poor. Preventative strategies for each of these groups will be considered separately here.

Adults

Most adult survivors of in-hospital cardiac arrest have a witnessed and monitored ventricular fibrillation (VF) arrest and are defibrillated immediately. The underlying cause of arrest in this group is usually primary myocardial ischaemia and an irritable myocardium. In comparison, cardiac arrest in patients in unmonitored ward areas is usually a predictable event not caused by primary cardiac disease. In this group, arrest often follows a period of slow and progressive physiological deterioration involving unrecognised or inadequately treated hypoxaemia and hypotension. The underlying cardiac arrest rhythm is usually asystole or PEA, and the chance of survival to hospital discharge is extremely poor.

Regular monitoring and early, effective treatment of seriously ill patients appear to improve clinical outcomes and prevent some cardiac arrests. Closer attention to patients who suffer a 'false' cardiac arrest may also improve outcome, as up to one third of these patients die during their in-hospital stay.

Deficiencies in acute care
Analysis of the critical events preceding many adult cardiac arrests demonstrates many significant antecedents, usually related to abnormalities of the airway, breathing, and circulation.[2] Often, medical and nursing staff do not possess acute-care knowledge and skills[3] and may lack confidence when dealing with acute-care problems. Specific areas of concern involve the incorrect use of oxygen therapy and a failure to monitor patients or to involve experienced senior staff in the immediate care of sick patients. Additional factors include a failure to use a systematic approach to the assessment of critically ill patients, poor communication, lack of teamwork, and insufficient use of treatment limitation plans.

Hospital processes may also have significant effects on patient outcome. For example, patients who are discharged from intensive care units (ICU) to general wards at night have an increased risk of in-hospital death compared to those discharged during the day and those discharged to high-dependency units. Higher nurse-patient staffing ratios are also associated with reduction in cardiac arrest rates, as well as rates of pneumonia, shock, and death.

Recognition of 'at-risk', or critically ill, adult patients

When patients deteriorate, they display common signs that represent failing respiratory, cardiovascular, and neurological systems. This is the basis for monitoring patients' vital signs. Abnormal physiology is common on general wards,[4] yet the important physiological observations of sick patients are measured and recorded less frequently than is desirable. Monitoring the respiratory rate is essential, as it may predict cardiorespiratory arrest.

In recent years, early warning scores (EWS), or 'calling-criteria' have been adopted by many hospitals to assist in the early detection of critical illness.[5] EWS systems allocate points to routine vital sign measurements on the basis of their deviation from an arbitrarily agreed 'normal' range. The weighted score of one or more vital sign observations, or more often the total EWS, is used to alert ward staff or critical care outreach teams to the deteriorating condition of the patient. Systems that incorporate 'calling-criteria' activate a response when one or more routinely measured physiological variables reach an extremely abnormal value. It might be supposed that a system that can track changes in physiology and warn of impending physiological collapse, rather than one that is triggered only when an extreme value of physiology has been reached, may detect acutely ill patients at an earlier stage.

The sensitivity, specificity, and accuracy of EWS or calling-criteria systems to identify sick patients have yet to be validated. Several studies have identified abnormalities of heart rate, blood pressure, respiratory rate, and conscious level as possible markers of impending critical events. However, as not all important vital signs are, or can be, recorded continuously in general ward areas, the ability of these systems to predict cardiac arrest remains unconfirmed. Gaps in vital sign data recording are common; the use of physiological systems can increase the frequency of vital sign monitoring. The medical and nursing response to a patient's abnormal physiology needs to be both appropriate and speedy, yet this is not always the case.

The clinical response

Traditionally, the response to cardiac arrest has been reactive, with a cardiac arrest team attending the patient after the cardiac arrest. The use of such teams appears to improve survival in circumstances where no coordinated cardiac arrest response previously existed. However, their impact in other settings is questionable. For example, in one study only patients who had return of spontaneous circulation before the cardiac arrest team arrived were alive at hospital discharge.[6] In some hospitals the role of the cardiac arrest team has been subsumed into that of the medical emergency team (MET). This team responds not only to cardiac arrests, but to patients with acute physiological deterioration. The MET usually comprises medical and nursing staff from intensive care and general medicine and responds to specific calling criteria. MET interventions often involve simple tasks such as starting oxygen therapy and intravenous fluids.

The results of research into the benefits of introducing a MET are variable. Studies with historical control groups show a reduction in cardiac arrests, deaths and unanticipated intensive care unit admissions, improved detection of medical errors, treatment-limitation decisions, and reduced postoperative ward deaths. A cluster-randomised controlled trial of the MET system demonstrated that the introduction of a MET increased the calling incidence for the team, but did not reduce the incidence of cardiac arrest, unexpected death, or unplanned ICU admission.[7]

In the UK, a system of pre-emptive ward care, based predominantly on individual or teams of nurses known as critical care outreach, has developed.[8] Although the data on the effects of outreach care are also inconclusive, it has been suggested that outreach teams may reduce ward deaths, postoperative adverse events, ICU admissions and readmissions, and increase survival.

The role of education in cardiac arrest prevention

The recognition that many cardiac arrests may be preventable has led to the development of postgraduate courses specifically designed to prevent physiological deterioration, critical illness, and cardiac arrest (e.g. Acute Life Threatening Events – Recognition and Treatment: ALERT).[9] Early evidence suggests that they can improve knowledge and change attitudes about acute care. Courses, such as Immediate Life Support and Advanced Life Support, now also include sections related to this important topic. Other courses focus on managing sick patients in the first 24 hours of critical illness when more direct critical care expertise is not immediately available. It is recognised that training in acute and critical care should commence early, and many countries have established curricula for inclusion in undergraduate medical education programmes.

Pregnant patients

The latest report of the triennial Confidential Enquiry into Maternal and Child Health (CEMACH) suggests that more than half of pregnancy-related deaths were associated with substandard care.[10] In general, these were caused by errors in diagnosis or patient treatment, or failure to refer to senior colleagues. Staff failed to recognise and act on the common signs of critical illness. There was also a lack of communication and clinical teamwork. The CEMACH report makes several recommendations to prevent deaths associated with pregnancy, including the need for hospitals to implement, audit, and regularly update multidisciplinary guidelines for the management of women at risk of, or who develop, complications in pregnancy. It also recommends that clinical protocols and local referral pathways, including patient transfer, should be developed for pregnant women with pre-existing medical conditions, a history of psychiatric illness, and serious complications of pregnancy (sepsis, pre-eclampsia and eclampsia, obstetric haemorrhage). The routine emergency 'fire drills' for maternal emergencies, including cardiopulmonary resuscitation, is emphasised.

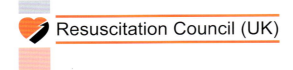
Resuscitation Council (UK)

Children

In children, cardiopulmonary arrest is more often due to profound hypoxaemia and hypotension than primary cardiac disease. Ventricular fibrillation is less common than asystole or pulseless electrical activity. As with adults, there may be opportunities to introduce strategies that will prevent arrest.

There is already evidence of marked, often untreated, abnormalities of common vital signs in the 24 hours prior to the admission of children to an ICU, similar to those reported in adults.[11] Recognition of the seriously ill child relies on determination of the normal and abnormal age-related values for vital signs, and reassessing them in the context of the progression of the child's condition. As in adults, serial measurement of heart rate, respiratory rate, temperature, blood pressure, and conscious level, particularly following any clinical intervention, must be performed and acted upon. Intervention at an early stage in an unwell child reduces significantly the risk of developing irreversible shock. Systemic blood pressure decreases at a late stage in shock in the child compared with the adult, and should not be used as the sole determinant of whether or not treatment is required.

Paediatric emergency teams, responding to early warning scores, have been established in some hospitals[12] and appear to reduce the incidence of cardiac arrest.

Resuscitation decisions

Cardiopulmonary resuscitation was originally conceived to save the lives of patients dying unexpectedly – 'hearts too young to die'. In-hospital death now invariably involves attempted cardiopulmonary resuscitation, even when the underlying condition and general health of the patient makes success unlikely – 'hearts too bad to live'. However, even when there is clear evidence that cardiac arrest or death are likely, ward staff rarely make decisions about the patient's resuscitation status. Improved knowledge, training, and do-not-attempt-resuscitation (DNAR) decision-making should improve patient care and prevent futile CPR attempts. Patients for whom cardiopulmonary resuscitation will not prolong life, and may merely prolong the dying process, should be identified early.

A DNAR decision should be considered when the patient:

- does not wish to have CPR, or
- will not survive cardiac arrest even if CPR is attempted.

Recommended strategies for the prevention of avoidable in-hospital cardiac arrests

1) Place critically ill patients, or those at risk of clinical deterioration, in areas where the level of care is matched to the level of patient sickness.

2) Regularly monitor such patients using simple vital sign observations (e.g. pulse, blood pressure, respiratory rate). Match the frequency and type of observations to the severity of illness of the patient.

3) Use an EWS system to identify patients who are critically ill, at risk of clinical deterioration or cardiopulmonary arrest, or both.

4) Use a patient vital signs chart that encourages and permits the regular measurement and recording of early warning scores.

5) Ensure that the hospital has a clear policy that requires a clinical response to deterioration in the patient's clinical condition. Provide advice on the further clinical management of the patient and the specific responsibilities of medical and nursing staff.

6) Introduce into each hospital a clearly identified response to critical illness. This will vary between sites, but may include an outreach service or clinical team (e.g. MET) capable of responding to acute clinical crises. This team should be alerted, using an early warning system, and the service must be available 24 hours a day.

7) Ensure that all clinical staff are trained in the recognition, monitoring, and management of the critically ill patient.

8) Agree a hospital DNAR policy, based on national guidelines, and ensure that it is understood by all clinical staff. Identify patients who do not wish to receive CPR and those for whom cardiopulmonary arrest is an anticipated terminal event for whom CPR would be inappropriate.

9) Audit all cardiac arrests, 'false arrests', unexpected deaths, and unanticipated intensive care unit admissions, using a common dataset. Audit the antecedents and clinical responses to these events.

References

1. Peberdy MA, Kaye W, Ornato JP, et al. Cardiopulmonary resuscitation of adults in the hospital: a report of 14720 cardiac arrests from the National Registry of Cardiopulmonary Resuscitation. Resuscitation 2003; 58: 297-308.

2. Kause J, Smith G, Prytherch D, et al. A comparison of antecedents to cardiac arrests, deaths and emergency intensive care admissions in Australia and New Zealand, and the United Kingdom--the ACADEMIA study. Resuscitation 2004; 62: 275-82.

3. Smith GB, Poplett N. Knowledge of aspects of acute care in trainee doctors. Postgrad Med J 2002; 78: 335-8.

4. Harrison GA, Jacques TC, Kilborn G, McLaws ML. The prevalence of recordings of the signs of critical conditions and emergency responses in hospital wards--the SOCCER study. Resuscitation 2005; 65: 149-57.

5. McArthur-Rouse F. Critical care outreach services and early warning scoring systems: a review of the literature. J.Adv.Nurs 2001; 36: 696-704.

6. Soar J, McKay U. A revised role for the hospital cardiac arrest team? Resuscitation 1998; 38: 145-9.

7. The MERIT study investigators. Introduction of the medical emergency team (MET) system: a cluster-randomised controlled trial. Lancet 2005; 365: 2091-7.

8. Priestley G, Watson W, Rashidian A, et al. Introducing Critical Care Outreach: a ward-randomised trial of phased introduction in a general hospital. Intensive Care Med 2004; 30: 1398-404.

9. Smith GB, Osgood VM, Crane S. ALERT™ - a multiprofessional training course in the care of the acutely ill adult patient. Resuscitation 2002; 52: 281-286.

10. Department of Health, Welsh Office, Scottish Office Department of Health, Department of Health and Social Services, Northern Ireland. Why mothers die. Report on confidential enquiries into maternal deaths in the United Kingdom, 2000-2002. London: The Stationery Office; 2004.

11. Tume L. A 3-year review of emergency PICU admissions from the ward in a specialist cardio-respiratory centre. Care of the Critically ill 2005; 21: 4-7.

12. Haines C. Acutely ill children within ward areas – care provision and possible development strategies. Nursing in Critical Care 2005; 10: 98-104.

In-hospital Resuscitation

Introduction

This new section in the guidelines describes the sequence of actions for starting in-hospital resuscitation. Hospital staff are often trained in basic life support (BLS) techniques that are more appropriate for the single lay rescuer in an out-of-hospital environment. These new guidelines are aimed primarily at healthcare professionals who are first to respond to an in-hospital cardiac arrest. Some of the guidelines are also applicable to healthcare professionals in other clinical settings.

The Royal College of Anaesthetists, the Royal College of Physicians of London, the Intensive Care Society, and the Resuscitation Council (UK) published a joint statement in 2004, *Cardiopulmonary resuscitation - standards for clinical practice and training.*[1] This document provides healthcare institutions with guidance on delivering an effective resuscitation service.

After in-hospital cardiac arrest the division between basic life support and advanced life support is arbitrary; in practice, the resuscitation process is a continuum and is based on common sense. The public expect that clinical staff should be able to undertake cardiopulmonary resuscitation (CPR). For all in-hospital cardiac arrests, ensure that:

- cardiorespiratory arrest is recognised immediately;

- help is summoned using a standard telephone number (e.g. 2222);

- CPR is started immediately using airway adjuncts, for example a pocket mask, and, if indicated, defibrillation attempted as soon as possible (within 3 min at the most).

Sequence for 'collapsed' patient in a hospital

1   **Ensure personal safety.**

2   **Check the patient for a response.**
- When a healthcare professional sees a patient collapse, or finds a patient apparently unconscious in a clinical area, he should first shout for help, then assess if the patient is responsive by gently shaking his shoulders and asking loudly, 'Are you all right?'

- If other members of staff are nearby it will be possible to undertake actions simultaneously.

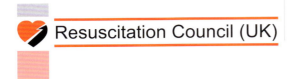
Resuscitation Council (UK)

In-hospital resuscitation

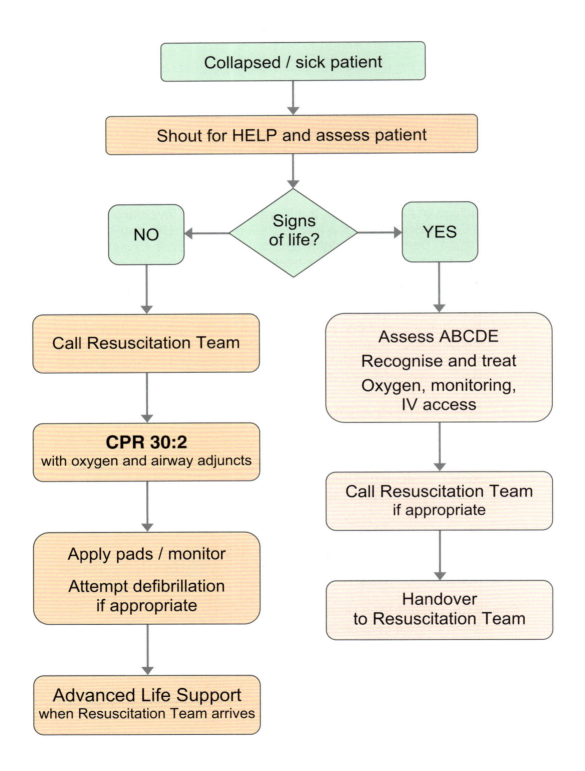

Collapsed / sick patient

Shout for HELP and assess patient

Signs of life?

NO

YES

Call Resuscitation Team

CPR 30:2
with oxygen and airway adjuncts

Apply pads / monitor

Attempt defibrillation
if appropriate

Advanced Life Support
when Resuscitation Team arrives

Assess ABCDE
Recognise and treat
Oxygen, monitoring,
IV access

Call Resuscitation Team
if appropriate

Handover
to Resuscitation Team

3 A   If the patient responds:

- Urgent medical assessment is required. Depending on the local protocols this may be by a resuscitation team (e.g. medical emergency team (MET)).

- While awaiting this team, assess the patient using the ABCDE approach.

- Give the patient oxygen.

- Attach monitoring leads.

- Obtain venous access.

3 B   If the patient does not respond:

- Shout for help (if this has not already been done).

- Turn the patient onto his back.

- Open the airway using head tilt and chin lift.

- Look in the mouth. If a foreign body or debris is visible, attempt to remove it, using suction or forceps as appropriate.

- If there is a risk of cervical spine injury, establish a clear upper airway by using jaw thrust or chin lift in combination with manual in-line stabilisation (MILS) of the head and neck by an assistant (if sufficient staff are available). If life-threatening airway obstruction persists despite effective application of jaw thrust or chin lift, add head tilt a small amount at a time until the airway is open; establishing a patent airway takes priority over concerns about a potential cervical spine injury.

- Keeping the airway open, look, listen, and feel for no more than **10 sec** to determine if the victim is breathing normally:
    - Listen at the victim's mouth for breath sounds.
    - Look for chest movement.
    - Feel for air on your cheek.

- Those experienced in clinical assessment may wish to assess the carotid pulse for not more than 10 sec. This may be performed simultaneously with checking for breathing or after the breathing check.

The exact sequence will depend on the training of staff and their experience in assessment of breathing and circulation. Agonal breathing (occasional gasps, slow, laboured, or noisy breathing) is common in the early stages of cardiac arrest - it is a sign of cardiac arrest and should not be mistaken for a sign of life.

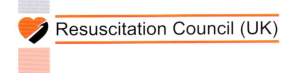

4 A   If the patient has a pulse or other signs of life:

- Urgent medical assessment is required. Depending on the local protocols this may take the form of a resuscitation team.

- While awaiting this team, assess the patient using the ABCDE approach.

- Give the patient oxygen.

- Attach monitoring.

- Insert an intravenous cannula.

4 B   If there is <u>no</u> pulse or other signs of life:

- One person should start CPR as others call the resuscitation team and collect the resuscitation equipment and a defibrillator. If only one member of staff is present, this will mean leaving the patient.

- Give 30 chest compressions followed by 2 ventilations.

- The correct hand position for chest compression is the middle of the lower half of the sternum. The recommended depth of compression is 4 to 5 cm and the rate is 100 compressions min^{-1}.

- Maintain the airway and ventilate the lungs with the most appropriate equipment immediately at hand. A pocket mask, which may be supplemented with an oral airway, is usually readily available. Alternatively, use a laryngeal mask airway (LMA) and self-inflating bag, or bag-mask, according to local policy. Tracheal intubation should be attempted only by those who are trained and experienced in this skill.

- Use an inspiratory time of 1 sec and give enough volume to produce chest rise as in normal breathing. Add supplemental oxygen as soon as possible.

- Once the patient's airway has been secured, continue chest compression uninterrupted (except for defibrillation or pulse checks when indicated) at a rate of 100 min^{-1}, and ventilate the lungs at approximately 10 breaths min^{-1}. Avoid hyperventilation.

- If there is no airway and ventilation equipment available, give mouth-to-mouth ventilation. If there are clinical reasons to avoid mouth-to-mouth contact, or you are unwilling or unable to do this, give chest compressions alone until help or airway equipment arrives. A pocket mask should be rapidly available in all clinical areas.

- When the defibrillator arrives, apply the electrodes to the patient and analyse the rhythm. The use of adhesive electrode pads or the 'quick-look' paddles technique will enable rapid assessment of heart rhythm compared with attaching ECG electrodes.

- If self-adhesive defibrillation pads are available, and there is more than one rescuer, apply the pads without interrupting chest compression. Pause briefly to assess the heart rhythm. If indicated, attempt either manual or automated external defibrillation.

- Recommence chest compressions immediately after the defibrillation attempt. Do not pause to assess the pulse or heart rhythm. Minimise interruptions to chest compression.

- Continue resuscitation until the resuscitation team arrives or the patient shows signs of life. If using an automated external defibrillator (AED), follow the voice prompts; if using a manual defibrillator follow the algorithm for advanced life support (ALS) (see adult ALS section).

- Once resuscitation is underway, and if there are sufficient people available, prepare intravenous cannulae and drugs likely to be used by the resuscitation team (e.g. adrenaline).

- Identify one person to be responsible for handover to the resuscitation team leader. Locate the patient's records.

- Change the person providing chest compression about every 2 min to prevent fatigue.

4 C   If the patient is <u>not</u> breathing but <u>has a pulse</u> (respiratory arrest):
- Ventilate the patient's lungs (as described above) and check for a pulse every 10 breaths (about every minute).

Only those confident in assessing breathing and a pulse will be able to make this diagnosis. If there are any doubts about the presence of a pulse, start chest compression and continue until more experienced help arrives.

5   If the patient has a monitored and witnessed cardiac arrest:
- Confirm cardiac arrest and shout for help.

- If a defibrillator is not immediately to hand consider giving a single precordial thump immediately after confirmation of VF/VT cardiac arrest. The precordial thump should be given only by healthcare professionals trained in the technique.

- If the initial rhythm is VF/VT and a defibrillator is immediately available, give a shock first.

- Start CPR immediately after the shock is delivered as described above.

- Continue resuscitation in accordance with the ALS algorithm (see adult ALS section).

Background notes

Sequence of actions

The exact sequence of actions after in-hospital cardiac arrest depends on several factors including:
- location (clinical or non-clinical area; monitored or unmonitored patients);
- skills of staff who respond;

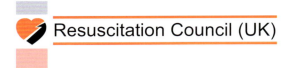

- number of responders;
- equipment available;
- hospital system for response to cardiac arrest and medical emergencies (e.g. MET, cardiac arrest team).

Location

Patients who have monitored arrests are usually diagnosed rapidly. Ward patients may have had a period of deterioration and an unwitnessed arrest. Ideally, all patients who are at high risk of cardiac arrest should be cared for in a monitored area where facilities for immediate resuscitation are available. Patients, visitors, or staff may also have a cardiac arrest in non-clinical areas (e.g. car parks, corridors).

Training

All healthcare professionals should be able to recognise cardiac arrest, call for help, and start resuscitation. Staff should do what they have been trained to do. For example, staff in critical care and emergency medicine may have more advanced resuscitation skills than staff who are not involved regularly in resuscitation in their normal clinical role. Hospital staff who attend a cardiac arrest may have different competencies in managing the airway, breathing, and circulation. Rescuers must undertake only the skills in which they are competent.

Trained healthcare staff cannot reliably assess breathing and pulse to confirm cardiac arrest.[2,3] Only those who are trained and experienced in pulse assessment should use pulse checks in addition to assessment of signs of life for confirmation of cardiac arrest. If the patient has no signs of life (based on lack of movement, breathing, or coughing), start CPR and continue until more experienced help arrives or the patient shows signs of life.

In Guidelines 2000 a method was recommended for finding the correct hand position for chest compression by placing one finger on the lower end of the sternum and sliding the other hand down to it. It has been shown that the same hand position can be found more quickly if rescuers are taught to 'place the heel of your hand in the centre of the chest with the other hand on top', provided the teaching includes a demonstration of placing the hands in the middle of the lower half of the sternum.[4]

The quality of chest compression during in-hospital CPR is frequently sub-optimal.[5] The team leader should monitor the quality of CPR and change rescuers if it is poor. The person doing chest compression will get tired. If there are enough rescuers this person should change about every 2 min.

The Resuscitation Council (UK) Immediate Life Support Course trains healthcare professionals in the skills required to start resuscitation, including defibrillation, and to be members of a cardiac arrest team.[6] The ALS Course teaches the skills required for leading a resuscitation team.[7,8]

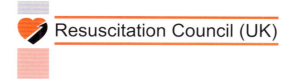
Resuscitation Council (UK)

Number of responders

The single responder must ensure that help is on its way. If other staff are nearby, several actions can be undertaken simultaneously.

Equipment available

All clinical areas should have immediate access to resuscitation equipment and drugs to facilitate rapid resuscitation of the patient in cardiopulmonary arrest. Ideally, the equipment used for resuscitation (including defibrillators) and the layout of equipment and drugs should be standardised throughout the hospital.[1]

Resuscitation team

The resuscitation team may take the form of a traditional cardiac arrest team, which is called only when cardiac arrest is recognised. Alternatively, hospitals may have strategies to recognise patients at risk of cardiac arrest and summon a team (e.g. MET) before cardiac arrest occurs.[9-11] The term 'resuscitation team' reflects the range of response teams. In-hospital cardiac arrests are rarely sudden or unexpected. A strategy of recognising patients at risk of cardiac arrest may enable some of these arrests to be prevented, or may prevent futile resuscitation attempts in those patients who are unlikely to benefit from CPR (See prevention of in-hospital cardiac arrest and decisions about cardiopulmonary resuscitation section).

References

1.	Gabbott D, Smith G, Mitchell S, et al. Cardiopulmonary resuscitation standards for clinical practice and training in the UK. Resuscitation 2005;64:13-9.

2.	Ruppert M, Reith MW, Widmann JH, et al. Checking for breathing: evaluation of the diagnostic capability of emergency medical services personnel, physicians, medical students, and medical laypersons. Ann Emerg Med 1999;34:720-9.

3.	Perkins GD, Stephenson B, Hulme J, Monsieurs KG. Birmingham assessment of breathing study (BABS). Resuscitation 2005;64:109-13.

4.	Handley AJ. Teaching hand placement for chest compression - a simpler technique. Resuscitation 2002; 53:29-36.

5.	Abella BS, Alvarado JP, Myklebust H, et al. Quality of cardiopulmonary resuscitation during in-hospital cardiac arrest. JAMA 2005;293:305-10.

6.	Soar J, Perkins GD, Harris S, Nolan JP. The immediate life support course. Resuscitation 2003;57:21-6.

7.	Nolan J. Advanced life support training. Resuscitation 2001;50:9-11.

8. Perkins G, Lockey A. The advanced life support provider course. BMJ 2002;325:S81.

9. Bellomo R, Goldsmith D, Uchino S, et al. A prospective before-and-after trial of a medical emergency team. Med J Aust 2003;179:283-7.

10. The MERIT study investigators. Introduction of the medical emergency team (MET) system: a cluster-randomised controlled trial. Lancet 2005;365:2091-7.

11. Kenward G, Castle N, Hodgetts T, Shaikh L. Evaluation of a medical emergency team one year after implementation. Resuscitation 2004;61:257-63.

Resuscitation Council (UK)

Adult Advanced Life Support

Introduction

This section on adult advanced life support (ALS) adheres to the same general principles as in Guidelines 2000, but incorporates some important changes. The guidelines in this section apply to healthcare professionals trained in ALS techniques. Laypeople, first responders, and automated external defibrillator (AED) users are referred to the basic life support (BLS) and AED sections.

Guideline changes

CPR before defibrillation

- In the case of out-of-hospital cardiac arrest attended, but unwitnessed, by healthcare professionals equipped with manual defibrillators, give CPR for 2 min (i.e. about 5 cycles at 30:2) before defibrillation.

- Do not delay defibrillation if an out-of-hospital arrest is witnessed by a healthcare professional.

- Do not delay defibrillation for in-hospital cardiac arrest.

Defibrillation strategy

- Treat ventricular fibrillation/pulseless ventricular tachycardia (VF/VT) with a single shock, followed by immediate resumption of CPR (30 compressions to 2 ventilations). Do not reassess the rhythm or feel for a pulse. After 2 min of CPR, check the rhythm and give another shock (if indicated).

- The recommended initial energy for biphasic defibrillators is 150-200 J. Give second and subsequent shocks at 150-360 J.

- The recommended energy when using a monophasic defibrillator is 360 J for both the initial and subsequent shocks.

Fine VF

- If there is doubt about whether the rhythm is asystole or fine VF, do NOT attempt defibrillation; instead, continue chest compression and ventilation.

Adrenaline (epinephrine)

VF/VT
- Give adrenaline 1 mg IV if VF/VT persists after a second shock.
- Repeat the adrenaline every 3-5 min thereafter if VF/VT persists.

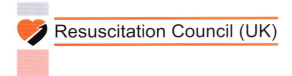

Resuscitation Council (UK)

Adult Advanced Life Support Algorithm

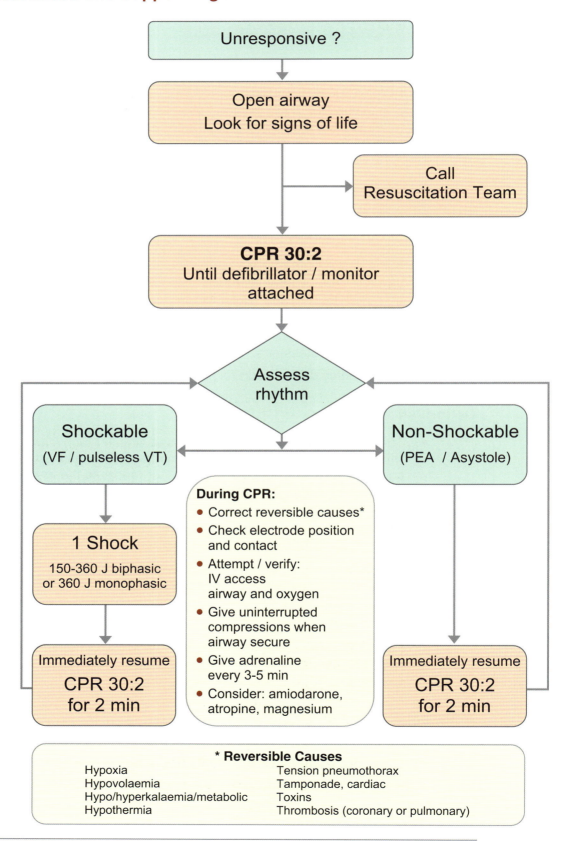

Unresponsive ?

↓

Open airway
Look for signs of life

→ Call
Resuscitation Team

↓

CPR 30:2
Until defibrillator / monitor
attached

↓

Assess
rhythm

Shockable
(VF / pulseless VT)

Non-Shockable
(PEA / Asystole)

1 Shock

150-360 J biphasic
or 360 J monophasic

↓

Immediately resume
CPR 30:2
for 2 min

Immediately resume
CPR 30:2
for 2 min

During CPR:
- Correct reversible causes*
- Check electrode position
  and contact
- Attempt / verify:
  IV access
  airway and oxygen
- Give uninterrupted
  compressions when
  airway secure
- Give adrenaline
  every 3-5 min
- Consider: amiodarone,
  atropine, magnesium

* Reversible Causes

Hypoxia	Tension pneumothorax
Hypovolaemia	Tamponade, cardiac
Hypo/hyperkalaemia/metabolic	Toxins
Hypothermia	Thrombosis (coronary or pulmonary)

Pulseless electrical activity / asystole

- Give adrenaline 1 mg IV as soon as intravenous access is achieved and repeat every 3-5 min.

Anti-arrhythmic drugs

- If VF/VT persists after three shocks, give amiodarone 300 mg by bolus injection. A further dose of 150 mg may be given for recurrent or refractory VF/VT, followed by an infusion of 900 mg over 24 h.

- If amiodarone is not available, lidocaine 1 mg kg^{-1} may be used as an alternative, but do not give lidocaine if amiodarone has already been given. Do not exceed a total dose of 3 mg kg^{-1} during the first hour.

Post resuscitation care – therapeutic hypothermia

- Unconscious adult patients with spontaneous circulation after out-of-hospital VF cardiac arrest should be cooled to 32-34°C for 12-24 h.

- Mild hypothermia may also benefit unconscious patients with spontaneous circulation after out-of-hospital cardiac arrest due to a non-shockable rhythm, or after cardiac arrest in hospital.

ALS treatment algorithm

Arrhythmias associated with cardiac arrest are divided into two groups: shockable rhythms (VF/VT) and non-shockable rhythms (asystole and PEA). The principle difference in management is the need for attempted defibrillation in patients with VF/VT. Subsequent actions, including chest compression, airway management and ventilation, venous access, administration of adrenaline, and the identification and correction of reversible factors, are common to both groups. The ALS treatment algorithm provides a standardised approach to the management of adult patients in cardiac arrest.

Shockable rhythms (VF/VT)

Sequence of actions

- Attempt defibrillation (one shock - 150-200 J biphasic or 360 J monophasic).

- Immediately resume chest compressions (30:2) without reassessing the rhythm or feeling for a pulse.

- Continue CPR for 2 min, then pause briefly to check the monitor:
  - If VF/VT persists:
    - Give a further (2nd) shock (150-360 J biphasic or 360 J monophasic).
    - Resume CPR immediately and continue for 2 min.
    - Pause briefly to check the monitor.

- If VF/VT persists give adrenaline 1 mg IV followed immediately by a (3rd) shock (150-360 J biphasic or 360 J monophasic).
- Resume CPR immediately and continue for 2 min.
- Pause briefly to check the monitor.
- If VF/VT persists give amiodarone 300 mg IV followed immediately by a (4th) shock (150-360 J biphasic or 360 J monophasic).
- Resume CPR immediately and continue for 2 min.
- Give adrenaline 1 mg IV immediately before alternate shocks (i.e. approximately every 3-5 min).
- Give a further shock after each 2 min period of CPR and after confirming that VF/VT persists.
  - If organised electrical activity is seen during this brief pause in compressions, check for a pulse.
    - If a pulse is present, start post-resuscitation care.
    - If no pulse is present, continue CPR and switch to the non-shockable algorithm.
  - If asystole is seen, continue CPR and switch to the non-shockable algorithm.

Precordial thump

Consider giving a single precordial thump when cardiac arrest is confirmed rapidly after a witnessed and monitored sudden collapse, and a defibrillator is not immediately to hand. A precordial thump should be undertaken immediately after confirmation of cardiac arrest but only by healthcare professionals trained in the technique. Using the ulnar edge of a tightly clenched fist, deliver a sharp impact to the lower half of the sternum from a height of about 20 cm, then retract the fist immediately to create an impulse-like stimulus. A precordial thump is most likely to be successful in converting VT to sinus rhythm. Successful treatment of VF by precordial thump is much less likely: in all the reported successful cases the precordial thump was given within the first 10 seconds of VF. There are very rare reports of a precordial thump converting a perfusing to a non-perfusing rhythm.

Explanation for the changes in the treatment of VF/VT

CPR before defibrillation

Although Guidelines 2000 recommended immediate defibrillation for all shockable rhythms, recent evidence indicates that a period of CPR before defibrillation may improve survival after prolonged collapse (> 5 min).[1] The duration of collapse is frequently difficult to estimate accurately, so give CPR before attempted defibrillation outside hospital, unless the arrest is witnessed by a healthcare professional or an AED is being used. This advice does NOT apply to lay responders using an AED outside hospital, who should apply the AED as soon as it is available.

In contrast, there is no evidence to support or refute CPR before defibrillation for in-hospital cardiac arrest. For this reason, after in-hospital VF/VT cardiac arrest, give a shock as soon as possible.

Defibrillation strategy

There are no published human or experimental studies comparing a single shock protocol with a three-stacked shock protocol for the treatment of VF/VT cardiac arrest. Experimental studies show that relatively short interruptions in chest compression to deliver rescue breaths or perform rhythm analysis are associated with reduced survival.[2,3] Interruptions in chest compression also reduce the chances of converting VF to another rhythm.[4] Significant interruptions in chest compression are common during out-of-hospital and in-hospital cardiac arrest.[5,6] When using a three-shock protocol, the time taken to deliver shocks and analyse the rhythm causes significant interruptions in CPR. This fact, combined with the improved first shock efficacy (for termination of VF/VT) of biphasic defibrillators, has prompted the recommendation of a single-shock strategy.

With first shock efficacy of biphasic waveforms exceeding 90%, failure to terminate VF/VT successfully implies the need for a period of CPR (to improve myocardial oxygenation) rather than a further shock. Even if defibrillation is successful in restoring a perfusing rhythm, it is very rare for a pulse to be palpable immediately afterwards, and the delay in trying to palpate a pulse will further compromise the myocardium if a perfusing rhythm has not been restored.[7] If a perfusing rhythm has been restored, giving chest compression does not increase the chance of VF recurring. In the presence of post-shock asystole, however, chest compressions may induce VF.

The initial shock from a biphasic defibrillator should be no lower than 120 J for rectilinear biphasic waveforms, and 150 J for biphasic truncated exponential waveforms. For uniformity, it is recommended that the initial biphasic shock should be at least 150 J. If an initial shock has been unsuccessful it may be worth attempting the second and subsequent shocks with a higher energy level. However, there is no evidence to support either a fixed or escalating energy protocol. Both strategies are acceptable. Manufacturers should display the effective waveform energy range on the face of the biphasic device. If you are unaware of the effective energy range of the device, use 200 J for the first shock. This 200 J default has been chosen because it falls within the reported range of selected energy levels that are effective for first and subsequent biphasic shocks, and can be provided by every biphasic manual defibrillator available today. It is a consensus default and not a recommended ideal. If biphasic devices are clearly labelled, and providers are familiar with the devices they use in clinical care, there will be no need for the default 200 J. Ongoing research is necessary to establish the most appropriate initial settings for both monophasic and biphasic defibrillators.

Because of the lower efficacy of monophasic defibrillators for terminating VF/VT, and the change to a single-shock strategy, the recommended initial energy level for the first shock using a monophasic defibrillator is 360 J. If needed, second and subsequent shocks should be given at 360 J. A monophasic waveform is less efficient than a biphasic waveform at terminating VF/VT, and most manufacturers now sell only biphasic devices. The urgency with which monophasic defibrillators are replaced must be determined locally, taking into consideration available resources and competing healthcare demands.

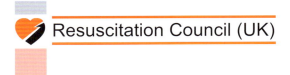

Fine VF

Fine VF that is difficult to distinguish from asystole is very unlikely to be shocked successfully into a perfusing rhythm. Continuing good quality CPR may improve the amplitude and frequency of the VF and improve the chance of successful defibrillation to a perfusing rhythm. Delivering repeated shocks in an attempt to defibrillate what is thought to be fine VF will increase myocardial injury, both directly from the electric current and indirectly from the interruptions in coronary blood flow.

Adrenaline

There is no placebo-controlled study that shows that the routine use of any vasopressor at any stage during human cardiac arrest increases survival to hospital discharge. Current evidence is insufficient to support or refute the routine use of any particular drug or sequence of drugs. Despite the lack of human data the use of adrenaline is still recommended, based largely on experimental data. The alpha-adrenergic actions of adrenaline cause vasoconstriction, which increases myocardial and cerebral perfusion pressure during cardiac arrest.

Immediate resumption of CPR after shock delivery, along with the elimination of a rhythm check at this stage, makes it difficult to select an ideal point in the ALS algorithm at which to give adrenaline. The consensus recommendation is to give adrenaline immediately after confirmation of the rhythm and just before shock delivery (**drug–shock–CPR–rhythm check** sequence). Have the adrenaline ready to give so that the delay between stopping chest compression and delivery of the shock is minimised. The adrenaline that is given immediately before the shock will be circulated by the CPR that follows the shock.

When the rhythm is checked 2 min after giving a shock, if a non-shockable rhythm is present and the rhythm is organised (complexes appear regular or narrow), try to palpate a pulse. Rhythm checks must be brief, and pulse checks undertaken only if an organised rhythm is observed. If an organised rhythm is seen during a 2-min period of CPR, do not interrupt chest compressions to palpate a pulse unless the patient shows signs of life suggesting return of spontaneous circulation (ROSC). If there is any doubt about the existence of a pulse in the presence of an organised rhythm, resume CPR. If the patient has ROSC, begin post-resuscitation care.

If the patient's rhythm changes to asystole or PEA see non-shockable rhythms below. In patients in asystole or PEA, give adrenaline 1 mg IV immediately intravenous access is achieved.

In both VF/VT and PEA / asystole, give adrenaline 1 mg IV every 3-5 min (approximately every other two-minute loop).

In patients with a spontaneous circulation, doses considerably smaller than 1 mg IV may be required to maintain an adequate blood pressure.

Vasopressin

A recent meta-analysis of five randomised trials showed no statistically significant difference between vasopressin and adrenaline for ROSC, death within 24 h, or death before hospital discharge.[8] A subgroup analysis, based on initial cardiac rhythm, did not show any statistically significant difference in the rate of death before hospital discharge. Despite the absence of placebo-controlled trials, adrenaline has been the standard vasopressor in cardiac arrest. There is insufficient evidence to support or refute the use of vasopressin as an alternative to, or in combination with, adrenaline in any cardiac arrest rhythm. Thus, adrenaline remains the primary vasopressor for the treatment of cardiac arrest in all rhythms.

Anti-arrhythmic drugs

There is no evidence that giving any anti-arrhythmic drug routinely during human cardiac arrest increases survival to hospital discharge. In comparison with placebo and lidocaine, the use of amiodarone in shock-refractory VF improves survival to hospital admission.[9,10] There are no data on the use of amiodarone for shock-refractory VF/VT when single shocks are used. On the basis of expert consensus, if VF/VT persists after three shocks, give amiodarone 300 mg by bolus injection during the brief rhythm analysis before delivery of the fourth shock. A further dose of 150 mg may be given for recurrent or refractory VF/VT, followed by an infusion of 900 mg over 24 h. Lidocaine 1 mg kg^{-1} may be used as an alternative if amiodarone is not available, but do not give lidocaine if amiodarone has been given already.

Non-shockable rhythms (PEA and asystole)

Pulseless electrical activity (PEA) is defined as cardiac electrical activity in the absence of any palpable pulse. These patients often have some mechanical myocardial contractions but they are too weak to produce a detectable pulse or blood pressure. PEA may be caused by reversible conditions that can be treated if they are identified and corrected (see below). Survival following cardiac arrest with asystole or PEA is unlikely unless a reversible cause can be found and treated effectively.

Sequence of actions for PEA

- Start CPR 30:2.
- Give adrenaline 1 mg IV as soon as intravascular access is achieved.
- Continue CPR 30:2 until the airway is secured, then continue chest compressions without pausing during ventilation.
- Recheck the rhythm after 2 min.
    - If there is no change in the ECG appearance:
        - Continue CPR.
        - Recheck the rhythm after 2 min and proceed accordingly.
        - Give further adrenaline 1 mg IV every 3-5 min (alternate loops).
    - If the ECG **changes** and organised electrical activity is seen, check for a pulse.

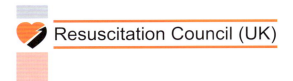
- If a pulse is present, start post-resuscitation care.
- If **no** pulse is present:
  - Continue CPR.
  - Recheck the rhythm after 2 min and proceed accordingly.
  - Give further adrenaline 1 mg IV every 3-5 min (alternate loops).

Sequence of actions for asystole and slow PEA (rate < 60 min^{-1})

- Start CPR 30:2.
- Without stopping CPR, check that the leads are attached correctly.
- Give adrenaline 1 mg IV as soon as intravascular access is achieved.
- Give atropine 3 mg IV (once only).
- Continue CPR 30:2 until the airway is secured, then continue chest compression without pausing during ventilation.
- Recheck the rhythm after 2 min and proceed accordingly.
- If VF/VT recurs, change to the shockable rhythm algorithm.
- Give adrenaline 1 mg IV every 3-5 min (alternate loops).

Asystole

Asystole is a condition that can be precipitated or exacerbated by excessive vagal tone. Theoretically, this can be reversed by a vagolytic drug; therefore, give atropine 3 mg (the dose that will provide maximum vagal blockade) for asystole or slow PEA (rate < 60 min^{-1}).

Whenever a diagnosis of asystole is made, check the ECG carefully for the presence of P waves because the patient may respond to cardiac pacing. There is no value in attempting to pace true asystole.

During CPR

During the treatment of persistent VF/VT or PEA / asystole, there should be an emphasis on giving good quality chest compression between defibrillation attempts, recognising and treating reversible causes (4 Hs and 4 Ts), and obtaining a secure airway and intravenous access. Healthcare providers must practise efficient coordination between CPR and shock delivery. The shorter the interval between cessation of chest compression and shock delivery, the more likely it is that the shock will be successful. Reduction in the interval from compression to shock delivery by even a few seconds can increase the probability of shock success. Providing CPR with a CV ratio of 30:2 is tiring; change the individual undertaking compressions every 2 min.

Potentially reversible causes

Potential causes or aggravating factors for which specific treatment exists must be sought during any cardiac arrest. For ease of memory, these are divided into two groups of four, based upon their initial letter, either H or T:

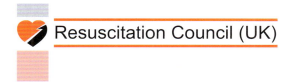

- **H**ypoxia
- **H**ypovolaemia
- **H**yperkalaemia, hypokalaemia, hypocalcaemia, acidaemia, and other metabolic disorders
- **H**ypothermia

- **T**ension pneumothorax
- **T**amponade
- **T**oxic substances
- **T**hromboembolism (pulmonary embolus/coronary thrombosis)

The four 'Hs'

Minimise the risk of **hypoxia** by ensuring that the patient's lungs are ventilated adequately with 100% oxygen. Make sure there is adequate chest rise and bilateral breath sounds. Using the techniques described below, check carefully that the tracheal tube is not misplaced in a bronchus or the oesophagus.

Pulseless electrical activity caused by **hypovolaemia** is usually due to severe haemorrhage. This may be precipitated by trauma, gastrointestinal bleeding, or rupture of an aortic aneurysm. Restore intravascular volume rapidly with fluid, coupled with urgent surgery to stop the haemorrhage.

Hyperkalaemia, hypokalaemia, hypocalcaemia, acidaemia, and other metabolic disorders are detected by biochemical tests or suggested by the patient's medical history, e.g. renal failure. A 12-lead ECG may be diagnostic. Intravenous calcium chloride is indicated in the presence of hyperkalaemia, hypocalcaemia, and calcium-channel-blocking drug overdose.

Suspect **hypothermia** in any drowning incident; use a low-reading thermometer.

The four 'Ts'

A **tension pneumothorax** may be the primary cause of PEA and may follow attempts at central venous catheter insertion. The diagnosis is made clinically. Decompress rapidly by needle thoracocentesis, and then insert a chest drain.

Cardiac **tamponade** is difficult to diagnose because the typical signs of distended neck veins and hypotension are usually obscured by the arrest itself. Cardiac arrest after penetrating chest trauma is highly suggestive of tamponade and is an indication for needle pericardiocentesis or resuscitative thoracotomy.

In the absence of a specific history, the accidental or deliberate ingestion of therapeutic or **toxic** substances may be revealed only by laboratory investigations. Where available, the appropriate antidotes should be used, but most often treatment is supportive.

The commonest cause of **thromboembolic** or mechanical circulatory obstruction is massive pulmonary embolus. If cardiac arrest is thought to be caused by pulmonary embolism, consider giving a thrombolytic drug immediately.

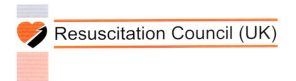
Thrombolysis may be considered in adult cardiac arrest, on a case-by-case basis, following initial failure of standard resuscitation in patients in whom an acute thrombotic aetiology for the arrest is suspected. Ongoing CPR is not a contraindication to thrombolysis.

Intravenous fluids

Hypovolaemia is a potentially reversible cause of cardiac arrest: infuse fluids rapidly if hypovolaemia is suspected. In the initial stages of resuscitation there are no clear advantages to using colloid: use saline or Hartmann's solution. Avoid dextrose; this is redistributed away from the intravascular space rapidly, and causes hyperglycaemia which may worsen neurological outcome after cardiac arrest.

Open-chest cardiac compression

Open-chest cardiac compression may be indicated for patients with cardiac arrest caused by trauma, in the early postoperative phase after cardiothoracic surgery, or when the chest or abdomen is already open, for example during surgery following trauma.

Signs of life

If signs of life (such as regular respiratory effort or movement) reappear during CPR, or readings from the patient's monitors (e.g. exhaled carbon dioxide or arterial blood pressure) are compatible with a return of spontaneous circulation, stop CPR and check the monitors briefly. If an organised cardiac rhythm is present, check for a pulse. If a pulse is palpable, continue post-resuscitation care, treatment of peri-arrest arrhythmias, or both. If no pulse is present, continue CPR.

Defibrillation

Strategies before defibrillation

Safe use of oxygen

In an oxygen-enriched atmosphere, sparks from poorly-applied defibrillator paddles can cause a fire. Taking the following precautions can minimise this risk:

- Remove any oxygen mask or nasal cannulae and place them at least 1 m away from the patient's chest.

- Leave the ventilation bag connected to the tracheal tube or other airway adjunct. Alternatively, disconnect the ventilation bag from the tracheal tube and move it at least 1 m from the patient's chest during defibrillation.

- The use of self-adhesive defibrillation pads, rather than manual paddles, may minimise the risk of sparks occurring.

Chest hair

It may be necessary rapidly to shave the area intended for electrode placement, but do not delay defibrillation if a razor is not immediately available.

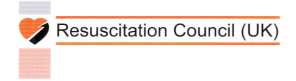

Paddle force

If using paddles, apply them firmly to the chest wall. The optimal force is 8 kg in adults, and 5 kg in children 1-8 years using adult paddles. Place water-based gel pads between the paddles and the patient's skin.

Electrode position

Place the right (sternal) electrode to the right of the sternum, below the clavicle. Place the apical paddle vertically in the mid-axillary line, approximately level with the V6 ECG electrode position or the female breast. This position should be clear of any breast tissue. It is important that this electrode is placed sufficiently laterally.

Antero-posterior electrode placement may be more effective than the traditional antero-apical position in cardioversion of atrial fibrillation. Either position is acceptable.

An implantable medical device (e.g. permanent pacemaker or automatic implantable cardioverter defibrillator (AICD)) may be damaged during defibrillation if current is discharged through electrodes placed directly over the device. Place the electrode away from the device or use an alternative electrode position. Remove any transdermal drug patches on the chest wall before defibrillation.

Pads versus paddles

Self-adhesive defibrillation pads are safe and effective and are an acceptable alternative to standard defibrillation paddles. They enable the operator to defibrillate from a safe distance, rather than leaning over the patient as occurs with paddles. When used for initial monitoring of a rhythm, both pads and paddles enable quicker delivery of the first shock compared with standard ECG electrodes, but pads are quicker than paddles.

Airway management and ventilation

The principles of airway and ventilation management remain unchanged from Guidelines 2000.

Patients requiring resuscitation often have an obstructed airway. Prompt assessment, with control of the airway and ventilation of the lungs, is essential. Without adequate oxygenation it may be impossible to restore a spontaneous cardiac output. In a witnessed cardiac arrest in the vicinity of a defibrillator, attempted defibrillation should take precedence over opening the airway.

Give high-flow oxygen. In the spontaneously breathing patient, masks with non-rebreathing reservoir bags are more effective than standard masks.

Basic airway manoeuvres and airway adjuncts

Assess the airway. Use head tilt and chin lift, or jaw thrust to open the airway. Simple airway adjuncts (oropharyngeal or nasopharyngeal airways) are often helpful, and sometimes essential, to maintain an open airway.

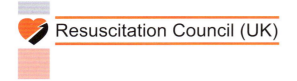

Ventilation

Provide artificial ventilation as soon as possible in any patient in whom spontaneous ventilation is inadequate or absent. Expired air ventilation (rescue breathing) is effective but the rescuer's expired oxygen concentration is only 16-17%, so it must be replaced as soon as possible by ventilation with oxygen-enriched air. A pocket resuscitation mask enables mouth-to-mask ventilation. Some enable supplemental oxygen to be given. Use a two-hand technique to maximise the seal with the patient's face. A self-inflating bag can be connected to a facemask, tracheal tube, or alternative airway device. The two-person technique for bag-mask ventilation is preferable. Deliver each breath over approximately 1 sec and give a volume that corresponds to normal chest movement; this represents a compromise between giving an adequate volume, minimising the risk of gastric inflation, and allowing adequate time for chest compression. During CPR with an unprotected airway, give two ventilations after each sequence of 30 chest compressions.

Once an airway device has been inserted, ventilate the lungs at a rate of about 10 breaths min^{-1} and continue chest compression without pausing during ventilation.

Alternative airway devices

Laryngeal mask airway (LMA)
A laryngeal mask airway is relatively easy to insert, and ventilation using an LMA is more efficient and easier than with a bag-mask. If gas leakage is excessive, chest compression will have to be interrupted to enable ventilation. Although an LMA does not protect the airway as reliably as a tracheal tube, pulmonary aspiration is uncommon when using an LMA during cardiac arrest.

The Combitube
A Combitube is relatively easy to insert and ventilation using this device is more efficient and easier than with a bag-mask. Great care must be taken to avoid attempting to ventilate the lungs through the wrong port of the Combitube.

Tracheal intubation

There is insufficient evidence to support or refute the use of any specific technique to maintain an airway and provide ventilation in adults with cardiopulmonary arrest. Despite this, tracheal intubation is perceived as the optimal method of providing and maintaining a clear and secure airway. It should be used only when trained personnel are available to carry out the procedure with a high level of skill and confidence.

The perceived advantages of tracheal intubation over bag-mask ventilation include:
- maintenance of a patent airway, which is protected from aspiration of gastric contents or blood from the oropharynx;
- ability to provide an adequate tidal volume reliably even when chest compressions are uninterrupted;

- the potential to free the rescuer's hands for other tasks;
- the ability to suction airway secretions;
- the provision of a route for giving drugs.

Use of the bag-mask is more likely to cause gastric distension which, theoretically, is more likely to cause regurgitation and aspiration. However, there are no reliable data to indicate that the incidence of aspiration is any higher in cardiac arrest patients ventilated using a bag-mask compared with those ventilated via a tracheal tube.

The perceived disadvantages of tracheal intubation over bag-mask ventilation include:

- the risk of an unrecognised, misplaced tracheal tube;
- a prolonged time without chest compression while intubation is attempted;
- a comparatively high failure rate.

Intubation success rates correlate with the intubation experience of the individual. Healthcare professionals who undertake intubation should do so only within a structured, monitored programme, which should include comprehensive competency-based training and regular opportunities to refresh skills.

Rescuers must weigh the risks and benefits of intubation against the need to provide effective chest compression. The intubation attempt will require interruption of chest compression, but once an advanced airway is in place ventilation can continue uninterrupted. Those skilled in advanced airway management should be able to undertake laryngoscopy without stopping chest compression; a brief pause in chest compression will be required as the tube is passed through the vocal cords. Alternatively, to avoid any interruption, the intubation attempt may be deferred until ROSC. No intubation attempt should take longer than 30 sec. If intubation has not been achieved by then, recommence bag-mask ventilation. After intubation, tube placement must be confirmed and the tube secured adequately.

Confirmation of correct placement of the tracheal tube

Unrecognised oesophageal intubation is the most serious complication of attempted tracheal intubation. Routine use of primary and secondary techniques to confirm correct placement of the tracheal tube should reduce this risk. Primary assessment should include bilateral observation of chest expansion, bilateral auscultation in the axillae (breath sounds should be equal and adequate), and auscultation over the epigastrium (breath sounds should not be heard). Clinical signs of correct tube placement (condensation in the tube, chest rise, breath sounds on auscultation of lungs, and inability to hear gas entering the stomach) are not completely reliable. Secondary confirmation of tracheal tube placement by an exhaled CO_2 or oesophageal detector device should reduce the risk of unrecognised oesophageal intubation. If there is doubt about correct tube placement, use the laryngoscope and look directly to see if the tube passes through the vocal cords.

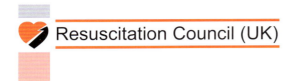

None of the secondary confirmation techniques will differentiate between a tube placed in a main bronchus and one placed correctly in the trachea. There are inadequate data to identify the optimal method of confirming tube placement during cardiac arrest, and all devices should be considered as adjuncts to other confirmatory techniques.

During cardiac arrest pulmonary blood flow may be so low that there is insufficient exhaled CO_2, so the CO_2 detector does not identify a correctly placed tracheal tube. When exhaled CO_2 is detected during cardiac arrest it indicates reliably that the tube is in the trachea or main bronchus, but when it is absent tracheal tube placement is best confirmed with an oesophageal detector device. A variety of electronic as well as simple, inexpensive, colorimetric CO_2 detectors are available for both in-hospital and out-of-hospital use.

Cricothyroidotomy

If it is impossible to ventilate an apnoeic patient with a bag-mask, or to pass a tracheal tube or alternative airway device, delivery of oxygen through a cannula or surgical cricothyroidotomy may be life saving.

Assisting the circulation

Intravenous access

Peripheral versus central venous drug delivery
Peripheral venous cannulation is quicker, easier to perform, and safer. Drugs injected peripherally must be followed by a flush of at least 20 ml of fluid. Central venous line insertion must cause minimal interruption of chest compression.

Intraosseous route
If intravenous access is difficult or impossible, consider the intraosseous route for both children and adults. The intraosseous route also enables withdrawal of marrow for venous blood gas analysis and measurement of electrolytes and haemoglobin concentration.

Tracheal route
If intravenous or intraosseous access cannot be established, some drugs can be given by the tracheal route. The dose of adrenaline is 3 mg diluted to at least 10 ml with sterile water.

Drugs

The use of adrenaline and anti-arrhythmic drugs has been discussed above.

Magnesium
Give magnesium sulphate 8 mmol (4 ml of a 50% solution) for refractory VF if there is any suspicion of hypomagnesaemia (e.g. patients on potassium-losing diuretics). Other indications are:

- ventricular tachyarrhythmias in the presence of possible hypomagnesaemia;
- torsade de pointes;
- digoxin toxicity.

Bicarbonate

Giving sodium bicarbonate routinely during cardiac arrest and CPR (especially in out-of-hospital cardiac arrest), or after ROSC, is not recommended. Give sodium bicarbonate (50 mmol) if cardiac arrest is associated with hyperkalaemia or tricyclic antidepressant overdose. Repeat the dose according to the clinical condition of the patient and the results of repeated blood gas analysis.

Atropine

Blockade of parasympathetic activity at both the sinoatrial (SA) node and the atrioventricular (AV) node may increase sinus automaticity and facilitate AV node conduction. The adult dose of atropine for asystole, or PEA with a rate < 60 min^{-1}, is 3 mg IV.

Calcium

Calcium is indicated during resuscitation from PEA if this is thought to be caused by:

- hyperkalaemia;
- hypocalcaemia;
- overdose of calcium-channel-blocking drugs;
- overdose of magnesium (e.g. during treatment of pre-eclampsia).

The initial dose of 10 ml 10% calcium chloride (6.8 mmol Ca^{2+}) may be repeated if necessary. Remember that calcium can slow the heart rate and precipitate arrhythmias. In cardiac arrest, calcium may be given by rapid intravenous injection. In the presence of a spontaneous circulation it should be given slowly. Do not give calcium solutions and sodium bicarbonate simultaneously by the same venous access.

Post-resuscitation care

Return of spontaneous circulation is just the first step towards the goal of complete recovery from cardiac arrest. Interventions in the post-resuscitation period influence the final outcome significantly. The post-resuscitation phase starts when ROSC is achieved. Once stabilised, the patient should be transferred to the most appropriate high-care area (e.g. intensive care unit or cardiac care unit) for continued monitoring and treatment.

Airway and breathing

Consider tracheal intubation, sedation, and controlled ventilation in any patient with obtunded cerebral function. Adjust ventilation to achieve normocarbia and monitor this using the end-tidal CO_2 and arterial blood gas values. Adjust the

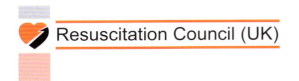
inspired oxygen concentrations to achieve adequate arterial oxygen saturation. Insert a gastric tube to decompress the stomach; gastric distension caused by mouth-to-mouth or bag-mask ventilation will splint the diaphragm and impair ventilation. Obtain a chest radiograph to check the position of the tracheal tube and central venous lines and exclude a pneumothorax associated with rib fractures from CPR.

Circulation

Haemodynamic instability is common after cardiac arrest. An arterial line for continuous blood pressure monitoring is essential, and the use of a non-invasive cardiac output monitor may be helpful. Infusion of fluids may be required to optimise filling. Conversely, diuretics and vasodilators may be needed to treat left ventricular failure. Infusion of an inotrope may be required to maintain a mean arterial blood pressure that is no lower than the normal pressure for the patient, and achieves an adequate urine output. Maintain the serum potassium concentration between 4.0-4.5 mmol l^{-1}. If there is evidence of coronary occlusion, consider the need for immediate revascularisation by thrombolytic therapy or percutaneous coronary intervention.

Disability (optimising neurological recovery)

Sedation
If sedation is required, short-acting drugs (e.g. propofol, alfentanil, remifentanil) will enable earlier neurological assessment.

Control of seizures
Seizures are relatively common in the post-resuscitation period and may cause cerebral injury. Control seizures with benzodiazepines, phenytoin, propofol, or a barbiturate as appropriate.

Temperature control
Treatment of hyperpyrexia
A period of hyperthermia is common in the first 48 h after cardiac arrest. The risk of a poor neurological outcome increases for each degree of body temperature above 37°C. Treat hyperthermia occurring in the first 72 h after cardiac arrest with antipyretics or active cooling.

Therapeutic hypothermia
Mild hypothermia is thought to suppress many of the chemical reactions associated with reperfusion injury. Two randomised clinical trials showed improved outcome in adults, remaining comatose after initial resuscitation from out-of-hospital VF cardiac arrest, who were cooled within minutes to hours after ROSC.[11,12]

Unconscious adult patients with spontaneous circulation after out-of-hospital VF cardiac arrest should be cooled to 32-34°C.[13] Cooling should be started as soon as possible and continued for at least 12-24 h. Induced hypothermia may also benefit unconscious adult patients with spontaneous circulation after out-of-hospital cardiac arrest from a non-shockable rhythm, or cardiac arrest in hospital. Treat shivering by ensuring adequate sedation and giving neuromuscular-blocking drugs. Bolus doses of neuromuscular blockers are usually adequate but infusions are occasionally necessary. Re-warm the patient slowly (0.25-0.5°C h^{-1}) and avoid hyperthermia. The optimum target temperature, rate of cooling, duration of hypothermia, and rate of rewarming have yet to be determined; further studies are essential.

External or internal cooling techniques or both can be used to initiate treatment. An infusion of 30 ml kg^{-1} saline at 4°C decreases core temperature by 1.5°C. Intravascular cooling enables more precise control of core temperature than external methods, but it is unknown whether this improves outcome.

Complications of mild therapeutic hypothermia include increased infection, cardiovascular instability, coagulopathy, hyperglycaemia, and electrolyte abnormalities such as hypophosphataemia and hypomagnesaemia.

Blood glucose control

There is a strong association between high blood glucose levels after resuscitation from cardiac arrest and poor neurological outcome. Tight control of blood glucose (4.4 - 6.1 mmol l^{-1}) using insulin reduces hospital mortality in critically ill adults, but this has not been demonstrated in post-cardiac-arrest patients specifically.

The optimal blood glucose target level in critically ill patients has not been determined. Comatose patients are at particular risk from unrecognised hypoglycaemia, and the risk of this complication occurring increases as the target blood glucose concentration is lowered.

In common with all critically ill patients, patients admitted to a critical-care environment after cardiac arrest should have their blood glucose monitored frequently and hyperglycaemia treated with an insulin infusion. The blood glucose concentration that triggers insulin therapy and the target range of blood glucose concentrations should be determined by local policy. There is a need for studies of glucose control after cardiac arrest.

Prognostication

There are no neurological signs that can predict outcome in the comatose patient in the first hours after ROSC. By three days after the onset of coma related to cardiac arrest, 50% of patients with no chance of ultimate recovery have died. In the remaining patients, the absence of pupil light reflexes on day three, and an absent motor response to pain on day three, are both independently predictive of a poor outcome (death or vegetative state) with very high specificity.

References

1.	Wik L, Hansen TB, Fylling F, et al. Delaying Defibrillation to Give Basic Cardiopulmonary Resuscitation to Patients with Out-of-Hospital Ventricular Fibrillation: A Randomized Trial. JAMA 2003;289:1389-95.

2.   Berg RA, Sanders AB, Kern KB, et al. Adverse hemodynamic effects of interrupting chest compressions for rescue breathing during cardiopulmonary resuscitation for ventricular fibrillation cardiac arrest. Circulation 2001;104:2465-70.

3.   Kern KB, Hilwig RW, Berg RA, Sanders AB, Ewy GA. Importance of continuous chest compressions during cardiopulmonary resuscitation: improved outcome during a simulated single lay-rescuer scenario. Circulation 2002;105:645-9.

4.   Eftestol T, Sunde K, Steen PA. Effects of interrupting precordial compressions on the calculated probability of defibrillation success during out-of-hospital cardiac arrest. Circulation 2002;105:2270-3.

5.   Wik L, Kramer-Johansen J, Myklebust H, et al. Quality of cardiopulmonary resuscitation during out-of-hospital cardiac arrest. JAMA 2005;293:299-304.

6.   Abella BS, Alvarado JP, Myklebust H, et al. Quality of cardiopulmonary resuscitation during in-hospital cardiac arrest. JAMA 2005;293:305-10.

7.   van Alem AP, Sanou BT, Koster RW. Interruption of cardiopulmonary resuscitation with the use of the automated external defibrillator in out-of-hospital cardiac arrest. Ann Emerg Med 2003;42:449-57.

8.   Aung K, Htay T. Vasopressin for cardiac arrest: a systematic review and meta-analysis. Arch Intern Med 2005;165:17-24.

9.   Kudenchuk PJ, Cobb LA, Copass MK, et al. Amiodarone for resuscitation after out-of-hospital cardiac arrest due to ventricular fibrillation. N Engl J Med 1999;341:871-8.

10.   Dorian P, Cass D, Schwartz B, Cooper R, Gelaznikas R, Barr A. Amiodarone as compared with lidocaine for shock-resistant ventricular fibrillation. N Engl J Med 2002;346:884-90.

11.   Hypothermia After Cardiac Arrest Study Group. Mild therapeutic hypothermia to improve the neurologic outcome after cardiac arrest. N Engl J Med 2002;346:549-56.

12.   Bernard SA, Gray TW, Buist MD, et al. Treatment of comatose survivors of out-of-hospital cardiac arrest with induced hypothermia. N Engl J Med 2002;346:557-63.

13.   Nolan JP, Morley PT, Vanden Hoek TL, Hickey RW. Therapeutic hypothermia after cardiac arrest. An advisory statement by the Advancement Life Support Task Force of the International Liaison committee on Resuscitation. Resuscitation 2003;57:231-5.

Peri-Arrest Arrhythmias

Introduction

Cardiac arrhythmias are well-recognised complications of myocardial infarction. They may precede ventricular fibrillation (VF) or follow successful defibrillation. The treatment algorithms described in this section have been designed to enable the non-specialist advanced life support (ALS) provider to treat the patient effectively and safely in an emergency; for this reason they have been kept as simple as possible. If patients are not acutely ill there may be several other treatment options, including the use of drugs (oral or parenteral) that will be less familiar to the non-expert. In this situation there will be time to seek advice from cardiologists or other senior doctors with the appropriate expertise.

Guideline changes

The principles of treating peri-arrest arrhythmias remain unchanged from Guidelines 2000. The bradycardia algorithm is virtually unchanged. Previous Resuscitation Council (UK) guidelines have included three separate tachycardia algorithms: broad-complex tachycardia, narrow-complex tachycardia, and atrial fibrillation. In the peri-arrest setting many treatment principles are common to all the tachycardias. For this reason, they have been combined into a single tachycardia algorithm.

Sequence of actions

In all cases, give oxygen and insert an intravenous cannula while the arrhythmia is assessed. Whenever possible, record a 12-lead ECG; this will help determine the precise rhythm, either before treatment or retrospectively, if necessary with the help of an expert. Correct any electrolyte abnormalities (e.g. K^+, Mg^{++}, Ca^{++}).

Assessment and treatment of all arrhythmias address two factors: the condition of the patient (stable versus unstable) and the nature of the arrhythmia.

Adverse signs

The presence or absence of adverse signs or symptoms will dictate the appropriate treatment for most arrhythmias. The following adverse factors indicate that a patient is unstable because of the arrhythmia:

Clinical evidence of low cardiac output

Pallor, sweating, cold, clammy extremities (increased sympathetic activity), impaired consciousness (reduced cerebral blood flow), and hypotension (e.g. systolic blood pressure < 90 mmHg).

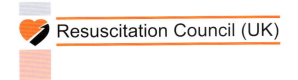

Resuscitation Council (UK)

Bradycardia Algorithm

(includes rates inappropriately slow for haemodynamic state)

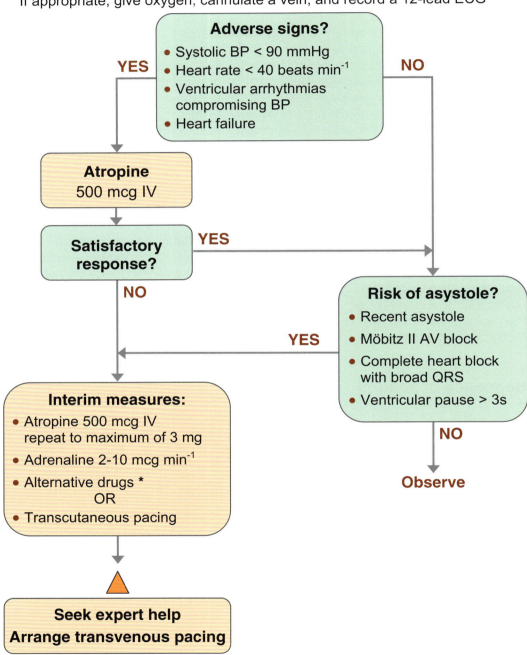

If appropriate, give oxygen, cannulate a vein, and record a 12-lead ECG

Adverse signs?
- Systolic BP < 90 mmHg
- Heart rate < 40 beats min^{-1}
- Ventricular arrhythmias compromising BP
- Heart failure

YES   **NO**

Atropine
500 mcg IV

Satisfactory response?   **YES**

NO

Risk of asystole?
- Recent asystole
- Möbitz II AV block
- Complete heart block with broad QRS
- Ventricular pause > 3s

YES

NO

Interim measures:
- Atropine 500 mcg IV repeat to maximum of 3 mg
- Adrenaline 2-10 mcg min^{-1}
- Alternative drugs *
  OR
- Transcutaneous pacing

Observe

Seek expert help
Arrange transvenous pacing

* Alternatives include:
    Aminophylline
    Isoprenaline
    Dopamine
    Glucagon (if beta-blocker or calcium-channel blocker overdose)
    Glycopyrrolate can be used instead of atropine

Excessive tachycardia

Very high heart rates (e.g. > 150 min^{-1}) reduce coronary blood flow and can cause myocardial ischaemia. Broad-complex tachycardias are tolerated by the heart less well than narrow-complex tachycardias.

Excessive bradycardia

This is defined as a heart rate of < 40 beats min^{-1}, but rates of < 60 beats min^{-1} may not be tolerated by patients with poor cardiac reserve.

Heart failure

Pulmonary oedema indicates failure of the left ventricle, and raised jugular venous pressure and hepatic engorgement indicate failure of the right ventricle.

Chest pain

The presence of chest pain implies that the arrhythmia, particularly a tachyarrhythmia, is causing myocardial ischaemia.

Treatment options

Having determined the rhythm and presence or absence of adverse signs, there are broadly three options for immediate treatment:

- anti-arrhythmic (and other) drugs;
- attempted electrical cardioversion;
- cardiac pacing.

Anti-arrhythmic drugs act more slowly and less reliably than electrical cardioversion in converting a tachycardia to sinus rhythm. Thus, drugs tend to be reserved for stable patients without adverse signs, and electrical cardioversion is usually the preferred treatment for the unstable patient displaying adverse signs.

Once an arrhythmia has been treated successfully, repeat the 12-lead ECG to enable detection of any underlying abnormalities that may require long-term therapy.

Bradycardia

Bradycardia is defined as a heart rate of < 60 beats min^{-1}. However, it is more helpful to classify a bradycardia as absolute (< 40 beats min^{-1}), or relative when the heart rate is inappropriately slow for the haemodynamic state of the patient.

The first step in the assessment of bradycardia is to determine if the patient is unstable. The following adverse signs may indicate instability:

- systolic blood pressure < 90 mm Hg;
- heart rate < 40 beats min^{-1};
- ventricular arrhythmias requiring suppression;
- heart failure.

Tachycardia Algorithm (with pulse)

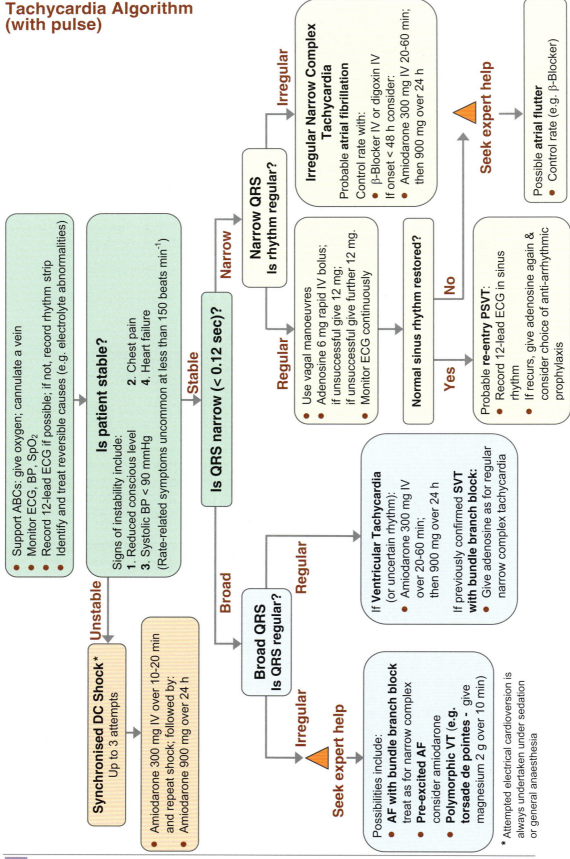

Support ABCs: give oxygen; cannulate a vein
- Monitor ECG, BP, SpO₂
- Record 12-lead ECG if possible; if not, record rhythm strip
- Identify and treat reversible causes (e.g. electrolyte abnormalities)

Is patient stable?

Signs of instability include:
1. Reduced conscious level
2. Chest pain
3. Systolic BP < 90 mmHg
4. Heart failure

(Rate-related symptoms uncommon at less than 150 beats min⁻¹)

Unstable

Synchronised DC Shock* Up to 3 attempts

- Amiodarone 300 mg IV over 10-20 min and repeat shock; followed by:
- Amiodarone 900 mg over 24 h

Stable

Is QRS narrow (< 0.12 sec)?

Broad — **Broad QRS Is QRS regular?**

Irregular — Seek expert help

Possibilities include:
- **AF with bundle branch block** treat as for narrow complex
- **Pre-excited AF** consider amiodarone
- **Polymorphic VT (e.g. torsade de pointes –** give magnesium 2 g over 10 min)

Regular

If **Ventricular Tachycardia** (or uncertain rhythm):
- Amiodarone 300 mg IV over 20-60 min; then 900 mg over 24 h

If previously confirmed **SVT with bundle branch block:**
- Give adenosine as for regular narrow complex tachycardia

Narrow — **Narrow QRS Is rhythm regular?**

Irregular — **Irregular Narrow Complex Tachycardia**

Probable atrial fibrillation

Control rate with:
- β-Blocker IV or digoxin IV

If onset < 48 h consider:
- Amiodarone 300 mg IV 20-60 min; then 900 mg over 24 h

Seek expert help → Possible **atrial flutter**
- Control rate (e.g. β-Blocker)

Regular

- Use vagal manoeuvres
- Adenosine 6 mg rapid IV bolus; if unsuccessful give 12 mg; if unsuccessful give further 12 mg.
- Monitor ECG continuously

Normal sinus rhythm restored?

Yes

Probable **re-entry PSVT**:
- Record 12-lead ECG in sinus rhythm
- If recurs, give adenosine again & consider choice of anti-arrhythmic prophylaxis

No → Seek expert help

* Attempted electrical cardioversion is always undertaken under sedation or general anaesthesia

If adverse signs are present, give atropine 500 microgram intravenously and, if necessary, repeat every 3 to 5 min, to a total of 3 mg. If a satisfactory response is achieved with atropine, or if the patient is stable, next determine if there is a risk of asystole, as indicated by:

- recent asystole;

- Möbitz type II AV block;

- complete (3rd degree) heart block (especially with broad QRS or initial heart rate less than 40 min^{-1});

- ventricular standstill of more than 3 sec.

Cardiac pacing is likely to be required if there is a risk of asystole or if the patient is unstable and has failed to respond satisfactorily to atropine. Under these circumstances the definitive treatment is transvenous pacing. One or more of the following interventions can be used to improve the patient's condition while waiting for the appropriate personnel and facilities:

- transcutaneous pacing;

- adrenaline infusion in the range of 2-10 microgram min^{-1} titrated against the response.

Other drugs that can be given for symptomatic bradycardia include dopamine, isoprenaline, and theophylline. Consider giving intravenous glucagon if beta-blockers or calcium-channel blockers are a potential cause of the bradycardia.

Complete heart block with a narrow QRS is not an absolute indication for pacing because atrioventricular junctional ectopic pacemakers (producing a narrow QRS) may provide a reasonable and stable heart rate.

Pacing

Transcutaneous pacing

Initiate transcutaneous pacing immediately if there is no response to atropine, if atropine is unlikely to be effective, or if the patient is severely symptomatic, particularly if there is high-degree AV block (Möbitz Type II $2°$ block or $3°$ block).

Fist pacing

If atropine is ineffective, and transcutaneous pacing is not immediately available, fist pacing can be attempted while waiting for pacing equipment: give serial rhythmic blows with the closed fist over the left lower edge of the sternum to pace the heart at a physiological rate of 50-70 min^{-1}.

Tachycardias

If the patient is unstable and deteriorating, with signs and symptoms caused by the tachycardia (e.g. impaired conscious level, chest pain, heart failure, hypotension, or other signs of shock), attempt synchronised cardioversion immediately. In patients with otherwise normal hearts, serious signs and symptoms are uncommon if the ventricular rate is < 150 min^{-1}. Patients with

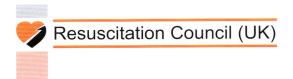
impaired cardiac function or significant co-morbidity may be symptomatic and unstable at lower heart rates. If cardioversion fails to restore sinus rhythm, and the patient remains unstable, give amiodarone 300 mg IV over 10 - 20 min and re-attempt electrical cardioversion. The loading dose of amiodarone can be followed by an infusion of 900 mg over 24 h.

Synchronised electrical cardioversion

For a broad-complex tachycardia or atrial fibrillation, start with 120-150 J biphasic shock (200 J monophasic) and increase in increments if this fails. Atrial flutter and regular narrow-complex tachycardia will often convert with lower energies: start with 70-120 J biphasic (100 J monophasic).

If a patient with tachycardia is stable (no serious signs or symptoms caused by the tachycardia), and is not deteriorating, there is time to evaluate the rhythm using the 12-lead ECG. Then determine treatment options and, if required, consult an expert. If the patient becomes unstable proceed immediately to synchronised electrical cardioversion. If a patient develops a tachyarrhythmia during, or as a complication of some other illness (e.g. infection, heart failure), treatment of the other medical problem is required also.

Broad-complex tachycardia

In broad-complex tachycardias the QRS complexes are ≥ 0.12 sec in duration, and are usually ventricular in origin. Broad-complex tachycardias may be caused also by supraventricular rhythms with aberrant conduction.

In the unstable periarrest patient assume that the rhythm is ventricular in origin and attempt electrical cardioversion. Conversely, if a patient with broad-complex tachycardia is stable, the next step is to determine if the rhythm is regular or irregular.

Regular broad-complex tachycardia

A regular broad-complex tachycardia is likely to be VT or a supraventricular rhythm with bundle branch block. In a stable patient, VT can be treated with amiodarone 300 mg intravenously over 20-60 minutes, followed by an infusion of 900 mg over 24 h. If a regular broad-complex tachycardia is known to be a supraventricular arrhythmia with bundle branch block, and the patient is stable, use the strategy indicated for narrow-complex tachycardia (below).

Irregular broad-complex tachycardia

This is most likely to be atrial fibrillation (AF) with bundle branch block, but careful examination of a 12-lead ECG (if necessary by an expert) may enable confident identification of the rhythm. Other possible causes are AF with ventricular pre-excitation (in patients with Wolff-Parkinson-White (WPW) syndrome), or polymorphic VT (e.g. torsade de pointes), but polymorphic VT is unlikely to be present without adverse features. Seek expert help with the assessment and treatment of irregular broad-complex tachyarrhythmia.

Treat torsade de pointes VT immediately by stopping all drugs known to prolong the QT interval. Correct electrolyte abnormalities, especially hypokalaemia. Give magnesium sulphate 2 g IV over 10 min. Obtain expert help, as other treatment (e.g. overdrive pacing) may be indicated to prevent relapse once the arrhythmia has been corrected. If adverse features develop, which is common, arrange immediate synchronised cardioversion. If the patient becomes pulseless, attempt defibrillation immediately (cardiac arrest algorithm).

Narrow-complex tachycardia

Regular narrow-complex tachycardias include:

- sinus tachycardia;
- AV nodal re-entry tachycardia (AVNRT) – the commonest type of regular narrow-complex tachyarrhythmia;
- AV re-entry tachycardia (AVRT) – due to WPW syndrome;
- atrial flutter with regular AV conduction (usually 2:1).

An irregular narrow-complex tachycardia is most likely to be atrial fibrillation (AF), or sometimes atrial flutter with variable AV conduction ('variable block').

Regular narrow-complex tachycardia

Sinus tachycardia
This is a common physiological response to a stimulus such as exercise or anxiety. In a sick patient it may occur in response to many stimuli such as pain, fever, anaemia, blood loss, and heart failure. Treatment is almost always directed at the underlying cause; trying to slow sinus tachycardia that has occurred in response to most of these situations will make the situation worse.

AVNRT and AVRT (paroxysmal supraventricular tachycardia)
AV nodal re-entry tachycardia is the commonest type of paroxysmal supraventricular tachycardia (PSVT), often seen in people without any other form of heart disease. It is relatively uncommon in the peri-arrest setting. It causes a regular, narrow-complex tachycardia, often with no clearly visible atrial activity on the ECG. The heart rate is commonly well above the typical range of sinus rhythm at rest (60-100 min^{-1}). It is usually benign, unless there is additional, co-incidental, structural heart disease or coronary disease, but it may cause symptoms that the patient finds frightening.

AV re-entry tachycardia occurs in patients with the WPW syndrome, and is also usually benign, unless there is additional structural heart disease. The common type of AVRT is a regular narrow-complex tachycardia, usually having no visible atrial activity on the ECG.

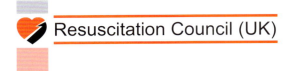

Atrial flutter with regular AV conduction (often 2:1 block)
This produces a regular narrow-complex tachycardia. It may be difficult to see
atrial activity and identify flutter waves in the ECG with confidence, so the rhythm
may be indistinguishable, at least initially, from AVNRT or AVRT.

Typical atrial flutter has an atrial rate of about 300 min^{-1}, so atrial flutter with 2:1
block produces a tachycardia of about 150 min^{-1}. Much faster rates (170 min^{-1} or
more) are unlikely to be caused by atrial flutter with 2:1 block.

Treatment of regular narrow-complex tachycardia
If the patient is unstable, with adverse features caused by the arrhythmia, attempt
synchronised electrical cardioversion. It is reasonable to give adenosine to an
unstable patient with a regular narrow-complex tachycardia while preparations
are being made for synchronised cardioversion. However, do not delay electrical
cardioversion if the adenosine fails to restore sinus rhythm.

In the absence of adverse features:
- Start with vagal manoeuvres. Carotid sinus massage or the Valsalva
  manoeuvre will terminate up to a quarter of episodes of paroxysmal
  SVT. Record an ECG (preferably multi-lead) during each manoeuvre.
  If the rhythm is atrial flutter, slowing of the ventricular response will
  often occur and reveal flutter waves.

- If the arrhythmia persists and is not atrial flutter, give adenosine 6 mg
  as a rapid intravenous bolus. Record an ECG (preferably multi-lead)
  during the injection. If the ventricular rate slows transiently, but the
  arrhythmia then returns, look for atrial activity, such as atrial flutter or
  other atrial tachycardia, and treat accordingly. If there is no response
  to adenosine 6 mg, give a 12 mg bolus. If there is no response give
  one further 12 mg bolus.

- Vagal manoeuvres or adenosine will terminate almost all AVNRT or
  AVRT within seconds. Failure to terminate a regular narrow-complex
  tachycardia with adenosine suggests an atrial tachycardia such as
  atrial flutter.

- If adenosine is contra-indicated, or fails to terminate a regular narrow
  complex tachycardia without demonstrating that it is atrial flutter, give
  a calcium-channel blocker, for example verapamil 2.5-5 mg
  intravenously over 2 min.

Irregular narrow-complex tachycardia

An irregular narrow-complex tachycardia is most likely to be AF with an
uncontrolled ventricular response or, less commonly, atrial flutter with variable AV
block. Record a 12-lead ECG to identify the rhythm. If the patient is unstable,
with adverse features caused by the arrhythmia, attempt synchronised electrical
cardioversion.

If there are no adverse features, treatment options include:
- rate control by drug therapy;
- rhythm control using drugs to encourage chemical cardioversion;

- rhythm control by electrical cardioversion;
- treatment to prevent complications (e.g. anticoagulation).

Obtain expert help to determine the most appropriate treatment for the individual patient. The longer a patient remains in AF the greater is the likelihood of atrial thrombus developing. In general, patients who have been in AF for more than 48 h should not be treated by cardioversion (electrical or chemical) until they have been fully anticoagulated for at least three weeks, or unless transoesophageal echocardiography has shown the absence of atrial thrombus.

If the aim is to control heart rate, options include a beta blocker, digoxin, magnesium, or combinations of these.

If the duration of AF is less than 48 h, and rhythm control is considered appropriate, this may be attempted using amiodarone (300 mg IV over 20-60 min followed by 900 mg over 24 h). Electrical cardioversion remains an option in this setting and will restore sinus rhythm in more patients than chemical cardioversion.

Seek expert help if any patient with AF is known or found to have ventricular pre-excitation (WPW syndrome). Avoid using adenosine, diltiazem, verapamil, or digoxin in patients with pre-excited AF or atrial flutter as these drugs block the AV node and cause a relative increase in pre-excitation.

Further reading

Blomstrom-Lundqvist C, Scheinman MM, Aliot EM et al. ACC/AHA/ESC Guidelines for the Management of Patients with Supraventricular Arrhythmias. European Heart Journal 2003; 24: 1857-1897.

Fuster V, Ryden LE, Asinger RW et al. ACC/AHA/ESC Guidelines for the Management of Patients with Atrial Fibrillation. European Heart Journal 2001; 22: 1852-1923.

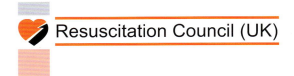
Resuscitation Council (UK)

Paediatric Basic Life Support

Introduction

The paediatric basic life support guidelines have been changed, partly in response to convincing new scientific evidence, and partly to simplify them in order to assist teaching and retention. As in the past, there remains a paucity of good quality evidence specifically on paediatric resuscitation, and some conclusions have had to be drawn from experimental work or extrapolated from adult data.

These guidelines have a strong focus on simplification, based on the knowledge that many children receive no resuscitation at all because rescuers fear doing harm as they have not been taught specific paediatric resuscitation. Consequently, a major area of discussion during the development of Guidelines 2005 has been the feasibility of applying the same guidelines to children as to adults.

Bystander resuscitation improves outcome significantly. There is good evidence from experimental models that doing either chest compression or expired air ventilation alone may result in a better outcome than doing nothing.[1] It follows that outcomes could be improved if bystanders who would otherwise do nothing, were encouraged to begin resuscitation, even if they do not follow an algorithm targeted specifically at children. There are, however, distinct differences between the predominantly adult arrest of cardiac origin and the asphyxial arrest which occurs commonly in children. Therefore, a separate paediatric algorithm is justified for healthcare professionals with a duty to respond to paediatric emergencies, who are in a position to receive enhanced training.

Guideline changes

Compression:ventilation ratios

- Lay rescuers should use a ratio of 30 compressions to 2 ventilations.
- Two or more rescuers with a duty to respond should use a ratio of 15 compressions to 2 ventilations.

Age definitions

- An infant is a child under 1 year.
- A child is between 1 year and puberty.

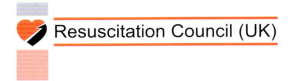

Paediatric Basic Life Support

**(Healthcare professionals
with a duty to respond)**

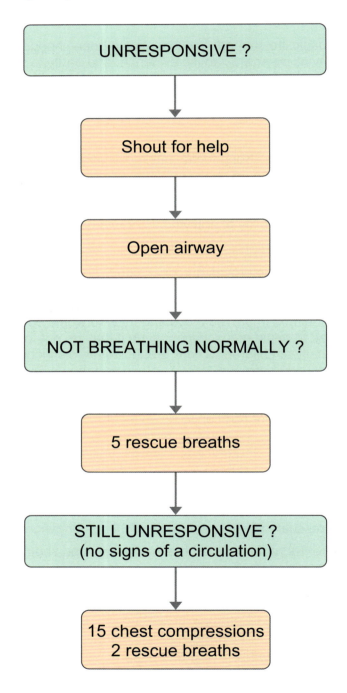

UNRESPONSIVE ?

↓

Shout for help

↓

Open airway

↓

NOT BREATHING NORMALLY ?

↓

5 rescue breaths

↓

STILL UNRESPONSIVE ?
(no signs of a circulation)

↓

15 chest compressions
2 rescue breaths

After 1 minute call resuscitation team then continue CPR

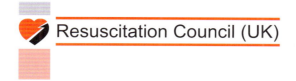

Automated external defibrillators

- A standard AED can be used in children over 8 years.

- Purpose-made paediatric pads, or programs which attenuate the energy output of an AED, are recommended for children between 1 and 8 years.

- If no such system or manually adjustable machine is available, an unmodified adult AED may be used for children older than 1 year.

- There is insufficient evidence to support a recommendation for or against the use of AEDs in children less than 1 year.

Foreign body airway obstruction sequence

- A simplified sequence of actions should be used for the management of foreign body airway obstruction (FBAO) in infants and children.

Infant and child BLS sequence

Rescuers who have been taught adult BLS, and have no specific knowledge of paediatric resuscitation, should use the adult sequence. The following modifications to the adult sequence will, however, make it more suitable for use in children:

- Give five initial rescue breaths before starting chest compression (adult sequence step 5B).

- If you are on your own, perform CPR for 1 min before going for help.

- Compress the chest by approximately one-third of its depth. Use two fingers for an infant and two hands for a child over 1 year, as needed to achieve an adequate depth of compression.

(See adult BLS section)

The following is the sequence that should be followed by healthcare professionals with a duty to respond to paediatric emergencies:

1   **Ensure the safety of rescuer and child.**

2   **Check the child's responsiveness:**
    - Gently stimulate the child and ask loudly, 'Are you all right?'
    - Do not shake infants, or children with suspected cervical spine injuries.

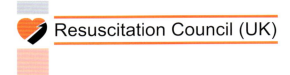

3 A   If the child responds by answering or moving:

- Leave the child in the position in which you find him (provided he is not in further danger).
- Check his condition and get help if needed.
- Reassess him regularly.

3 B   If the child does not respond:

- Shout for help.
- Open the child's airway by tilting the head and lifting the chin:
  - o With the child initially in the position in which you find him, place your hand on his forehead and gently tilt his head back.
  - o At the same time, with your fingertip(s) under the point of the child's chin, lift the chin. Do not push on the soft tissues under the chin as this may block the airway.
  - o If you still have difficulty in opening the airway, try the jaw thrust method: place the first two fingers of each hand behind each side of the child's mandible (jaw bone) and push the jaw forward. Both methods may be easier if the child is turned carefully onto his back.

If you suspect that there may have been an injury to the neck, try to open the airway using chin lift or jaw thrust alone. If this is unsuccessful, add head tilt a small amount at a time until the airway is open.

4   Keeping the airway open, look, listen, and feel for normal breathing by putting your face close to the child's face and looking along the chest:

- **Look** for chest movements.
- **Listen** at the child's nose and mouth for breath sounds.
- **Feel** for air movement on your cheek.

Look, listen, and feel for **no more** than **10 sec** before deciding that breathing is absent.

5 A   If the child is breathing normally:

- Turn the child onto his side into the recovery position (see below).
- Check for continued breathing.

5 B   If the child is not breathing or is making agonal gasps (infrequent, irregular breaths):

- Carefully remove any obvious airway obstruction.
- Give 5 initial rescue breaths.
- While performing the rescue breaths note any gag or cough response to your action. These responses, or their absence, will form part of your assessment of 'signs of a circulation', described below.

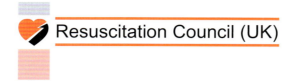

Rescue breaths for a child over 1 year:

- Ensure head tilt and chin lift.

- Pinch the soft part of his nose closed with the index finger and thumb of your hand on his forehead.

- Open his mouth a little, but maintain the chin upwards.

- Take a breath and place your lips around his mouth, making sure that you have a good seal.

- Blow steadily into his mouth over about 1-1.5 sec watching for chest rise.

- Maintaining head tilt and chin lift, take your mouth away from the victim and watch for his chest to fall as air comes out.

- Take another breath and repeat this sequence 5 times. Identify effectiveness by seeing that the child's chest has risen and fallen in a similar fashion to the movement produced by a normal breath.

Rescue breaths for an infant:

- Ensure a neutral position of the head and apply chin lift.

- Take a breath and cover the mouth and nasal apertures of the infant with your mouth, making sure you have a good seal. If the nose and mouth cannot both be covered in the older infant, the rescuer may attempt to seal only the infant's nose or mouth with his mouth (if the nose is used, close the lips to prevent air escape).

- Blow steadily into the infant's mouth and nose over 1-1.5 sec sufficient to make the chest visibly rise.

- Maintain head tilt and chin lift, take your mouth away from the victim, and watch for his chest to fall as air comes out.

- Take another breath and repeat this sequence 5 times.

If you have difficulty achieving an effective breath, the airway may be obstructed:

- Open the child's mouth and remove any visible obstruction. Do not perform a blind finger sweep.

- Ensure that there is adequate head tilt and chin lift but also that the neck is not over extended.

- If head tilt and chin lift has not opened the airway, try the jaw thrust method.

- Make up to 5 attempts to achieve effective breaths. If still unsuccessful, move on to chest compression.

6   Check for signs of a circulation (signs of life):

Take no more than 10 sec to:

- Look for signs of a circulation. These include any movement, coughing, or normal breathing (not agonal gasps - these are infrequent, irregular breaths).

- Check the pulse (if you are trained and experienced) **but ensure you take no more than 10 sec to do this:**
  - In **a child over 1 year** — feel for the carotid pulse in the neck.
  - In **an infant** — feel for the brachial pulse on the inner aspect of the upper arm.

7 A   If you are confident that you can detect signs of a circulation within 10 sec:
- Continue rescue breathing, if necessary, until the child starts breathing effectively on his own.
- Turn the child onto his side (into the recovery position) if he remains unconscious.
- Re-assess the child frequently.

7 B   If there are no signs of a circulation,
<u>or</u> no pulse,
<u>or</u> a slow pulse (less than 60 min^{-1} with poor perfusion),
<u>or</u> you are not sure:
- Start chest compression.
- Combine rescue breathing and chest compression.

For all children, compress the lower third of the sternum:
- To avoid compressing the upper abdomen, locate the xiphisternum by finding the angle where the lowest ribs join in the middle. Compress the sternum one finger's breadth above this.
- Compression should be sufficient to depress the sternum by approximately one-third of the depth of the chest.
- Release the pressure, then repeat at a rate of about 100 min^{-1}.
- After 15 compressions, tilt the head, lift the chin, and give two effective breaths.
- Continue compressions and breaths in a ratio of 15:2.

Lone rescuers may use a ratio of 30:2, particularly if they are having difficulty with the transition between compression and ventilation.

Although the rate of compressions will be 100 min^{-1}, the actual number delivered will be less than 100 because of pauses to give breaths. The best method for compression varies slightly between infants and children.

Chest compression in infants:
- The lone rescuer should compress the sternum with the tips of two fingers.
- If there are two or more rescuers, use the encircling technique:

> o   Place both thumbs flat, side by side, on the lower third of the sternum (as above), with the tips pointing towards the infant's head.
>
> o   Spread the rest of both hands, with the fingers together, to encircle the lower part of the infant's rib cage with the tips of the fingers supporting the infant's back.
>
> o   Press down on the lower sternum with your two thumbs to depress it approximately one-third of the depth of the infant's chest.

Chest compression in children over 1 year:

- Place the heel of one hand over the lower third of the sternum (as above).

- Lift the fingers to ensure that pressure is not applied over the child's ribs.

- Position yourself vertically above the victim's chest and, with your arm straight, compress the sternum to depress it by approximately one-third of the depth of the chest.

- In larger children, or for small rescuers, this may be achieved most easily by using both hands with the fingers interlocked.

8   Continue resuscitation until:

- the child shows signs of life (spontaneous respiration, pulse, movement);

- further qualified help arrives;

- you become exhausted.

When to call for assistance

It is vital for rescuers to get help as quickly as possible when a child collapses:

- When more than one rescuer is available, one starts resuscitation while another goes for assistance.

- If only one rescuer is present, undertake resuscitation for about **1 min** before going for assistance. To minimise interruptions in CPR, it may be possible to carry an infant or small child whilst summoning help.

- The only exception to performing 1 min of CPR before going for help is in the case of a child with a **witnessed, sudden** collapse when the rescuer is alone. In this case cardiac arrest is likely to be an arrhythmia and the child may need defibrillation. Seek help immediately if there is no one to go for you.

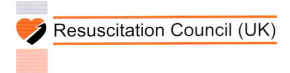
Resuscitation Council (UK)

Explanatory notes

Definitions

An **infant** is a child under 1 year.

A **child** is between 1 year and puberty. It is neither appropriate nor necessary to establish onset of puberty formally. If the rescuer believes the victim to be a child he should use the paediatric guidelines.

Compression:ventilation ratios

The publication, *2005 International Consensus on Cardiopulmonary Resuscitation and Emergency Cardiovascular Care Science with Treatment Recommendations* (CoSTR), recommends that the compression:ventilation ratio should be based on whether one or more rescuers are present. CoSTR also recommends that lay rescuers, who usually learn only single-rescuer techniques, should be taught to use a ratio of 30 compressions to 2 ventilations. This is the same ratio as recommended for adults and enables anyone trained in BLS techniques to resuscitate children with minimal additional information. Two or more rescuers with a duty to respond should learn a ratio with more rescue breaths (15:2), as this has been validated by experimental and mathematical studies.[2,3] This latter group, who would normally be healthcare professionals, should receive enhanced training targeted specifically at the resuscitation of children.

Although there are no data to support the superiority of any particular ratio in children, ratios of between 5:1 and 15:2 have been studied and there is increasing evidence that the 5:1 ratio delivers an inadequate number of compressions.[4,5] There is certainly no justification for having two separate ratios for children greater or less than 8 years, so a single ratio of 15:2 for multiple rescuers with a duty to respond is a logical simplification.

Although the CoSTR recommendation is based on the number of rescuers present, it would certainly negate the main benefit of simplicity if lay rescuers were taught a different ratio for use if there were two of them. Similarly, those with a duty to respond, who would normally be taught to use a ratio of 15:2, should not be compelled to use the 30:2 ratio if they are alone, unless they are not achieving an adequate number of compressions because of difficulty in the transition between ventilation and compression.

Age definitions

The adoption of a single compression:ventilation ratio for children of all ages, together with the change in advice on the lower age limit for the use of automated external defibrillators (AEDs), renders the Guidelines 2000 division between children above and below 8 years unnecessary. The differences between adult and paediatric resuscitation are largely based on differing aetiology, with primary cardiac arrest being more common in adults whereas children usually suffer from secondary cardiac arrest. The onset of puberty, which is the physiological end of childhood, is the most logical landmark for the upper age limit for use of paediatric guidelines. This has the advantage of being simple to determine in contrast to an age limit, as age may be unknown at the start of resuscitation.

Clearly, it is inappropriate and unnecessary to establish the onset of puberty formally; if the rescuer believes the victim to be a child then he should use the paediatric guidelines. If a misjudgment is made, and the victim turns out to be a young adult, little harm will accrue as studies of aetiology have shown that the paediatric pattern of arrest continues into early adulthood.

It is necessary to differentiate between infants and older children, as there are some important differences between these two groups.

Chest compression technique

The modification of age definitions enables a simplification of the advice on chest compression. The method for determining the landmarks for infant compression is now the same as that for older children, as there is evidence that the previous recommendation could result in compression over the upper abdomen.[6] Infant compression techniques remain the same: two-finger compression for single rescuers and two-thumb encircling technique for two or more rescuers. For older children there is no division between the one- or two-hand techniques;[7] the emphasis is on achieving an adequate depth of compression with minimal interruptions, using one or two hands according to rescuer preference.

Automated external defibrillators

Since Guidelines 2000 there have been case reports of safe and successful use of AEDs in children less than 8 years. Furthermore, recent studies have shown that AEDs are capable of identifying arrhythmias accurately in children and are extremely unlikely to advise a shock inappropriately. Consequently, advice on the use of AEDs has been revised to include all children greater than 1 year.[8] Nevertheless, if there is any possibility that an AED may need to be used in children, the purchaser should check that the performance of the particular model has been tested against paediatric arrhythmias.

Many manufacturers now supply purpose-made paediatric pads or programs which typically attenuate the output of the machine to 50-75 J.[9] These devices are recommended for children between 1 and 8 years. If no such system or manually adjustable machine is available, an unmodified adult AED may be used in children older than 1 year. There is currently insufficient evidence to support a recommendation for or against the use of AEDs in children less than 1 year.

Recovery position

An unconscious child whose airway is clear and who is breathing spontaneously should be turned onto his side into the recovery position. There are several recovery positions; each has its advocates. The important principles to be followed are:

- The child should be placed in as near a true lateral position as possible with his mouth dependant to enable free drainage of fluid.

- The position should be stable. In an infant, this may require the support of a small pillow or a rolled-up blanket placed behind his back to maintain the position.

- There should be no pressure on the chest that impairs breathing.

- It should be possible to turn the child onto his side and to return him back easily and safely, taking into consideration the possibility of cervical spine injury.

- The airway should be accessible and easily observed.

- The adult recovery position is suitable for use in children.

Foreign body airway obstruction (FBAO)

Recognition of FBAO

When a foreign body enters the airway the child reacts immediately by coughing in an attempt to expel it. A spontaneous cough is likely to be more effective and safer than any manoeuvre a rescuer might perform. However, if coughing is absent or ineffective, and the object completely obstructs the airway, the child will rapidly become asphyxiated. Active interventions to relieve FBAO are therefore required only when coughing becomes ineffective, but they then need to be commenced rapidly and confidently.

The majority of choking events in children occur during play or whilst eating, when a carer is usually present. Events are therefore frequently witnessed, and interventions are usually initiated when the child is conscious.

FBAO is characterised by the sudden onset of respiratory distress associated with coughing, gagging, or stridor. Similar signs and symptoms may also be associated with other causes of airway obstruction, such as laryngitis or epiglottitis, which require different management. Suspect FBAO if:

- the onset was very sudden;

- there are no other signs of illness;

- there are clues to alert the rescuer, for example a history of eating or playing with small items immediately prior to the onset of symptoms.

General signs of FBAO	
• Witnessed episode	
• Coughing or choking	
• Sudden onset	
• Recent history of playing with or eating small objects	
Ineffective coughing	**Effective cough**
• Unable to vocalise	• Crying or verbal response to questions
• Quiet or silent cough	• Loud cough
• Unable to breathe	• Able to take a breath before coughing
• Cyanosis	• Fully responsive
• Decreasing level of consciousness	

Relief of FBAO

Safety and summoning assistance

Safety is paramount. Rescuers should avoid placing themselves in danger and consider the safest action to manage the choking child:

- If the child is coughing effectively, then no external manoeuvre is necessary. Encourage the child to cough, and monitor continuously.
- If the child's coughing is, or is becoming, ineffective, **shout for help** immediately and determine the child's conscious level.

Conscious child with FBAO

- If the child is still conscious but has absent or ineffective coughing, give back blows.
- If back blows do not relieve the FBAO, give chest thrusts to infants or abdominal thrusts to children. These manoeuvres create an 'artificial cough' to increase intrathoracic pressure and dislodge the foreign body.

Back blows

In an infant:

- Support the infant in a head-downwards, prone position, to enable gravity to assist removal of the foreign body.
- A seated or kneeling rescuer should be able to support the infant safely across his lap.

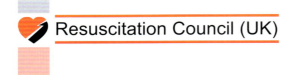
Resuscitation Council (UK)

Paediatric FBAO Treatment

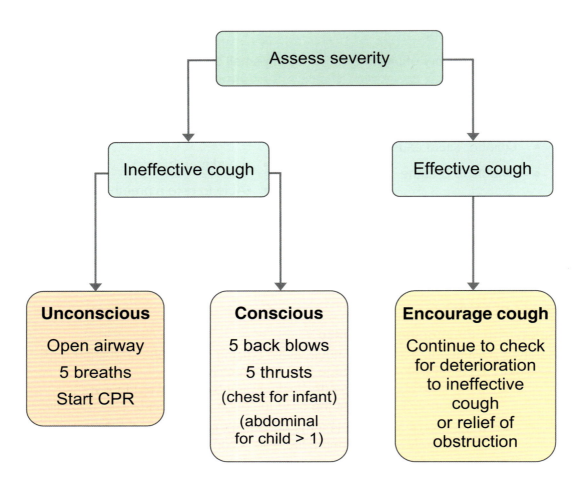

- Support the infant's head by placing the thumb of one hand at the angle of the lower jaw, and one or two fingers from the same hand at the same point on the other side of the jaw.
- Do not compress the soft tissues under the infant's jaw, as this will exacerbate the airway obstruction.
- Deliver up to 5 sharp back blows with the heel of one hand in the middle of the back between the shoulder blades.
- The aim is to relieve the obstruction with each blow rather than to give all 5.

In a child over 1 year:

- Back blows are more effective if the child is positioned head down.
- A small child may be placed across the rescuer's lap as with an infant.
- If this is not possible, support the child in a forward-leaning position and deliver the back blows from behind.

If back blows fail to dislodge the object, and the child is still conscious, use chest thrusts for infants or abdominal thrusts for children. **Do not use abdominal thrusts (Heimlich manoeuvre) for infants.**

Chest thrusts for infants:

- Turn the infant into a head-downwards supine position. This is achieved safely by placing your free arm along the infant's back and encircling the occiput with your hand.
- Support the infant down your arm, which is placed down (or across) your thigh.
- Identify the landmark for chest compression (lower sternum approximately a finger's breadth above the xiphisternum).
- Deliver 5 chest thrusts. These are similar to chest compressions, but sharper in nature and delivered at a slower rate.

Abdominal thrusts for children over 1 year:

- Stand or kneel behind the child. Place your arms under the child's arms and encircle his torso.
- Clench your fist and place it between the umbilicus and xiphisternum.
- Grasp this hand with your other hand and pull sharply inwards and upwards.
- Repeat up to 5 times.
- Ensure that pressure is not applied to the xiphoid process or the lower rib cage as this may cause abdominal trauma.

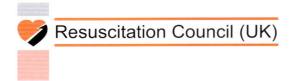

Following chest or abdominal thrusts, reassess the child:

- If the object has not been expelled and the victim is still conscious, continue the sequence of back blows and chest (for infant) or abdominal (for children) thrusts.
- Call out, or send, for help if it is still not available.
- Do not leave the child at this stage.

If the object is expelled successfully, assess the child's clinical condition. It is possible that part of the object may remain in the respiratory tract and cause complications. If there is any doubt, seek medical assistance. Abdominal thrusts may cause internal injuries and all victims so treated should be examined by a medical practitioner.

Unconscious child with FBAO

- If the child with FBAO is, or becomes, unconscious place him on a firm, flat surface.
- Call out, or send, for help if it is still not available.
- Do not leave the child at this stage.

Airway opening:

- Open the mouth and look for any obvious object.
- If one is seen, make an attempt to remove it with a single finger sweep.

Do not attempt blind or repeated finger sweeps - these can impact the object more deeply into the pharynx and cause injury.

Rescue breaths:

- Open the airway and attempt 5 rescue breaths.
- Assess the effectiveness of each breath: if a breath does not make the chest rise, reposition the head before making the next attempt.

Chest compression and CPR:

- Attempt 5 rescue breaths and if there is no response, proceed immediately to chest compression regardless of whether the breaths are successful.
- Follow the sequence for single rescuer CPR (step 7B above) for approximately 1 min before summoning EMS (if this has not already been done by someone else).
- When the airway is opened for attempted delivery of rescue breaths, look to see if the foreign body can be seen in the mouth.
- If an object is seen, attempt to remove it with a single finger sweep.

- If it appears that the obstruction has been relieved, open and check the airway as above. Deliver rescue breaths if the child is not breathing.

- If the child regains consciousness and is breathing effectively, place him in a safe side-lying (recovery) position and monitor breathing and conscious level whilst awaiting the arrival of EMS.

References

1. Berg RA, Hilwig RW, Kern KB, Babar I, Ewy GA. "Bystander" chest compressions and assisted ventilation independently improve outcome from piglet ashpyxial pulseless "cardiac arrest". Circulation 2000; 101:1743 – 1748.

2. Babbs CF, Nadkarni, V. Optimizing Chest Compression to Rescue Ventilation Ratios during One-rescuer CPR by Professionals and Lay Persons: Children are not just little adults. Resuscitation 2004; 61:173-81.

3. Berg RA, Hilwig RW, Kern KB, Babar I, Ewy GA. Simulated mouth-to-mouth ventilation and chest compressions (bystander cardiopulmonary resuscitation) improves outcome in a swine model of pre-hospital paedicatric asphyxial cardiac arrest. Crit Care Med 1999; 27:1893 –1899.

4. Dorph E, Wik L, Steen PA. Effectiveness of ventilation-compression ratios 1:5 and 2:15 in simulated single rescuer paediatric resuscitation. Resuscitation 2002; 54:259-64.

5. Whyte S, Wyllie JP. Paediatric basic life support a practical assessment. Resuscitation 1999; 41:153-157.

6. Clements F, McGowan J. Finger position for chest compressions in cardiac arrest in infants. Resuscitation 2000; 44:43-46.

7. Stevenson AG, McGowan J, Evans AL, Graham CA. CPR for children: one hand or two? Resuscitation 2005; 64: 205-8.

8. Samson R, Berg R, Bingham R and Pediatric Advanced Life Support Task Force, ILCOR. Use of automated external defibrillators for children: an update. An advisory statement from the Pediatric Advanced Life Support Task Force, International Liaison Committee on Resuscitation. Resuscitation 2003; 57: 237- 43.

9. Tang W, Weil MH, Jorgenson D, Klouche K, Morgan C, Yu T, Sun S, Snyder D. Fixed-energy biphasic waveform defibrillation in a pediatric model of cardiac arrest and resuscitation. Crit Care Med 2002; 30:2736-41.

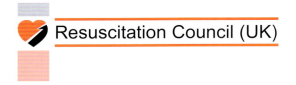

Resuscitation Council (UK)

Paediatric Advanced Life Support

Introduction

There is concern that resuscitation from cardiac arrest is not performed as well as it might because the variations in guidelines for different age groups cause confusion to providers, and therefore poor performance. Most of the changes in paediatric guidelines for 2005 have been made for simplification and to minimise differences between adult and paediatric protocols. It is hoped that this will assist teaching and retention. The guidelines have not, however, been simplified in the face of contradictory evidence or against an understanding of pathophysiology.

There remains a paucity of good quality evidence on which to base the resuscitation of infants and children. Most conclusions have had to be drawn from extrapolated adult studies and from experimental work.

Guideline Changes

- Where possible, give drugs intravascularly (intravenous or intraosseous), rather than by the tracheal route.

- Either uncuffed or cuffed tracheal tubes may be used in infants and children in the hospital setting.

- One defibrillating shock, rather than three 'stacked' shocks, is recommended for ventricular fibrillation/pulseless ventricular tachycardia (VF/VT).

- When using a manual defibrillator, the shock energy for children is 4 J kg^{-1} for all shocks.

- A standard AED can be used in children over 8 years.

- Purpose-made paediatric pads, or programs which attenuate the energy output of an AED, are recommended for children between 1 and 8 years.

- If no such system or manually adjustable machine is available, an unmodified adult AED may be used for children older than 1 year.

- There is insufficient evidence to support a recommendation for or against the use of AEDs in children less than 1 year.

- The dose of adrenaline (epinephrine) during cardiac arrest is 10 microgram kg^{-1} on each occasion.

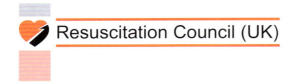

Paediatric Advanced Life Support

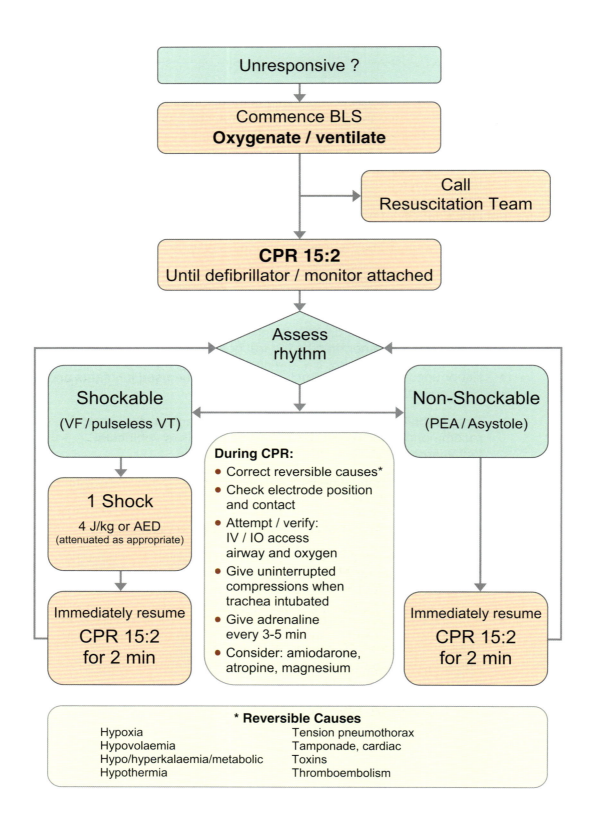

Unresponsive ?

Commence BLS
Oxygenate / ventilate

Call
Resuscitation Team

CPR 15:2
Until defibrillator / monitor attached

Assess rhythm

Shockable
(VF / pulseless VT)

Non-Shockable
(PEA / Asystole)

1 Shock
4 J/kg or AED
(attenuated as appropriate)

During CPR:
- Correct reversible causes*
- Check electrode position and contact
- Attempt / verify:
  IV / IO access
  airway and oxygen
- Give uninterrupted compressions when trachea intubated
- Give adrenaline every 3-5 min
- Consider: amiodarone, atropine, magnesium

Immediately resume
CPR 15:2
for 2 min

Immediately resume
CPR 15:2
for 2 min

* Reversible Causes

Hypoxia	Tension pneumothorax
Hypovolaemia	Tamponade, cardiac
Hypo/hyperkalaemia/metabolic	Toxins
Hypothermia	Thromboembolism

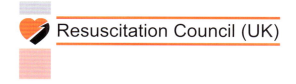 Resuscitation Council (UK)

Sequence of Actions

1   Establish basic life support.

2   Oxygenate, ventilate, and start chest compression:

- Provide positive-pressure ventilation with high-concentration inspired oxygen.

- Provide ventilation initially by bag and mask. Ensure a patent airway by using an airway manoeuvre as described in the paediatric basic life support section.

- As soon as is feasible, an experienced operator should intubate the child. This will both control the airway and enable chest compression to be given continuously, thus improving coronary perfusion pressure.

- Take care to ensure that ventilation remains effective when continuous chest compressions are started.

- Use a compression rate of 100 min^{-1}.

- Once the child has been intubated and compressions are uninterrupted, use a ventilation rate of approximately 10 min^{-1}.

3   Attach a defibrillator or monitor:

- Assess and monitor the cardiac rhythm.

- If using a defibrillator, place one defibrillator pad or paddle on the chest wall just below the right clavicle, and one in the left anterior axillary line.

- Pads or paddles for children should be 8 - 12 cm in size, and 4.5 cm for infants. In infants and small children it may be best to apply the pads or paddles to the front and back of the chest.

- Place monitoring electrodes in the conventional chest positions.

4   Assess rhythm and check for signs of a circulation (signs of life):

- Look for signs of a circulation, which include responsiveness, coughing, and normal breathing.

- Check the pulse if trained to do so:
    - **Child** – feel for the carotid pulse in the neck.
    - **Infant** – feel for the brachial pulse on the inner aspect of the upper arm.

- Take no more than 10 sec for the pulse check.

- Assess the rhythm on the monitor:
    - Non-shockable (asystole or pulseless electrical activity) **OR**
    - Shockable (VF/VT).

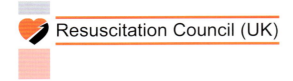

5 A   Non-shockable (asystole or pulseless electrical activity):
This is the more common finding in children.

- **Perform continuous CPR**:
    - Continue to ventilate with high-concentration oxygen.
    - If ventilating with bag-mask give 15 chest compressions to 2 ventilations for all ages.
    - If the patient is intubated, chest compressions can be continuous as long as this does not interfere with satisfactory ventilation.
    - Use a compression rate of 100 min^{-1}.
    - Once the child has been intubated and compressions are uninterrupted use a ventilation rate of approximately 10 min^{-1}.

Note: Once there is return of spontaneous circulation (ROSC) the ventilation rate should be 12 - 20 min^{-1}. Measure exhaled CO_2 to ensure correct tracheal tube placement.

- **Give adrenaline:**
    - If venous or intraosseous (IO) access has been established, give adrenaline 10 microgram kg^{-1} (0.1 ml kg^{-1} of 1 in 10,000 solution).
    - If there is no circulatory access, attempt to obtain IO access.
    - If circulatory access is not present, and cannot be quickly obtained, but the patient has a tracheal tube in place, consider giving adrenaline 100 microgram kg^{-1} via the tracheal tube (1 ml kg^{-1} of 1 in 10,000 or 0.1 ml kg^{-1} of 1 in 1,000 solution). This is the least satisfactory route (see routes of drug administration).

- **Continue CPR.**

- **Repeat the cycle:**
    - Give adrenaline 10 microgram kg^{-1} every 3 to 5 min, (i.e. every other loop), while continuing to maintain effective chest compression and ventilation without interruption. Unless there are exceptional circumstances, the dose should be 10 microgram kg^{-1} again for this and subsequent doses.
    - Once the airway is protected by tracheal intubation, continue chest compression without pausing for ventilation. Provide ventilation at a rate of 10 min^{-1} and compression at 100 min^{-1}.
    - When circulation is restored, ventilate the child at a rate of 12 - 20 breaths min^{-1} to achieve a normal pCO_2, and monitor exhaled CO_2.

- **Consider and correct reversible causes:**
  - o **H**ypoxia
  - o **H**ypovolaemia
  - o **H**yper/hypokalaemia (electrolyte disturbances)
  - o **H**ypothermia

  - o **T**ension pneumothorax
  - o **T**amponade
  - o **T**oxic/therapeutic disturbance
  - o **T**hromboembolism

- **Consider the use of other medications such as alkalising agents.**

5 B   Shockable (VF/VT)

This is less common in paediatric practice but likely when there has been a witnessed and sudden collapse. It is commoner in the intensive care unit and cardiac ward.

- **Defibrillate the heart:**
  - o Give 1 shock of 4 J kg^{-1} if using a manual defibrillator.
  - o If using an AED for a child of 1-8 years, deliver a paediatric-attenuated adult shock energy.
  - o If using an AED for a child over 8 years, use the adult shock energy.

- **Resume CPR:**
  - o Without reassessing the rhythm or feeling for a pulse, resume CPR **immediately,** starting with chest compression.

- **Continue CPR for 2 min.**

- **Pause briefly to check the monitor:**
  - o If still VF/VT, give a second shock at 4 J kg^{-1} if using a manual defibrillator, **OR** the adult shock energy for a child over 8 years using an AED, **OR** a paediatric-attenuated adult shock energy for a child between 1 year and 8 years .

- **Resume CPR immediately after the second shock.**

- **Consider and correct reversible causes (see above: 4Hs and 4Ts).**

- **Continue CPR for 2 min.**

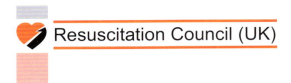

- **Pause briefly to check the monitor:**
  - o **If still VF/VT:**
    - Give adrenaline 10 microgram kg^{-1} followed immediately by a (3rd) shock.
    - Resume CPR immediately and continue for 2 min.

- **Pause briefly to check the monitor**.
  - o **If still VF/VT:**
    - Give an intravenous bolus of amiodarone 5 mg kg^{-1} and an immediate further (4th) shock.
    - Continue giving shocks every 2 min, minimising the breaks in chest compression as much as possible.
    - Give adrenaline immediately before every other shock (i.e. every 3-5 min) until return of spontaneous circulation (ROSC).

Note: After each 2 min of uninterrupted CPR, pause briefly to assess the rhythm.

  - o **If still VF/VT:**
    - Continue CPR with the shockable (VF/VT) sequence.

  - o **If asystole:**
    - Continue CPR and switch to the non-shockable (asystole or pulseless electrical activity) sequence as above.

  - o **If organised electrical activity is seen,** check for a pulse:
    - If there is ROSC, continue post-resuscitation care.
    - If there is **no** pulse, and there are no other signs of a circulation, give adrenaline 10 microgram kg^{-1} and continue CPR as for the non-shockable sequence as above.

Important note

Uninterrupted, good-quality CPR is vital. Chest compression and ventilation should be interrupted only for defibrillation. Chest compression is tiring for providers. The team leader should continuously assess and feed back on the quality of the compressions, and change the providers every 2 min.

Explanatory notes

Routes of drug administration

Studies in children and adults have shown that atropine, adrenaline, naloxone, lidocaine, and vasopressin are absorbed via the trachea, albeit resulting in lower blood concentrations than the same dose given intravascularly. However, experimental studies suggest that the lower adrenaline concentrations achieved in this way may produce transient beta-adrenergic effects. These effects can be detrimental, causing hypotension and lower coronary artery perfusion pressure, thereby reducing the likelihood of return of spontaneous circulation.[1] On the other hand, prospective, randomised trials in adults and children show that intraosseous access is safe and effective; practice indicates that this route is increasingly being used successfully.

Tracheal tubes

Several studies[2, 3] have shown no greater risk of complications for children less than 8 years when cuffed tracheal tubes rather than uncuffed tubes are used in the operating room and intensive care unit. Cuffed tracheal tubes are as safe as uncuffed tubes for infants (except newborns) and children if rescuers use the correct tube size and cuff inflation pressure, and verify tube position. Under certain circumstances (e.g. poor lung compliance, high airway resistance, and large glottic air leak) cuffed tracheal tubes may be preferable. Therefore, either uncuffed or cuffed tracheal tubes may be used in infants and children, but only in the hospital setting.

Shock sequence

For VF/VT, one defibrillating shock rather than three 'stacked' shocks is now recommended. This new recommendation for the sequence of defibrillation in children is based on extrapolated data from adult and experimental studies with biphasic devices. Evidence shows a high rate of success for first-shock conversion of ventricular fibrillation (VF).[4] Furthermore, interruption of chest compression reduces coronary perfusion pressure, myocardial viability, and the chance of successful defibrillation.

Shock energy level

The ideal energy level for safe and effective defibrillation in children is unknown. The recommendation of 2 - 4 J kg^{-1} in Guidelines 2000 was based on a single historical study of effective outcomes.

Extrapolation from adult data and experimental studies shows that biphasic shocks are at least as effective as monophasic shocks and produce less post-shock myocardial dysfunction. A few studies have shown that an initial monophasic or biphasic shock level of 2 J kg^{-1} generally terminates paediatric VF. Paediatric case series have reported that shock levels of more than 4 J kg^{-1} (up to 9 J kg^{-1}) have effectively defibrillated children less than 12 years with negligible adverse effects. In experimental studies, high energy levels cause less myocardial damage in young hearts than in adult hearts.[5-8]

A variable-dose manual defibrillator, or an AED able to recognise paediatric shockable rhythms and equipped with dose attenuation, is preferred in paediatric practice.

- Standard AEDs may be used in children over 8 years.

- Purpose-made paediatric pads, or devices/programs which attenuate the energy output of an AED, are recommended for children between 1 and 8 years.

- If no such system or manually adjustable machine is available, however, an unmodified adult AED may be used for children older than 1 year.

There is insufficient information to recommend for or against the use of an AED in infants less than one year. Manual defibrillation must be available for defibrillating infants.

Dose of adrenaline

In paediatric studies[9,10], no improvement in survival rates, and a trend towards worse neurological outcomes, have been shown after the administration of high-dose adrenaline during cardiac arrest. Children in cardiac arrest should, therefore, be given adrenaline 10 microgram kg^{-1} for the first and subsequent IV doses. Routine use of high-dose IV adrenaline (100 microgram kg^{-1}) is not recommended and may be harmful, particularly in asphyxial arrests. High-dose adrenaline should be considered only in exceptional circumstances, for example after beta-blocker overdose.

Drugs used in CPR

Adrenaline

This is an endogenous catecholamine with potent alpha, beta 1, and beta 2 adrenergic actions. Its use has never been subjected to trial in humans, but the drug still plays a major role in the treatment algorithms both for non-shockable and shockable cardiac arrest rhythms. This is supported by experimental studies and its known effect of improving relative coronary and cerebral perfusion.

Adrenaline induces vasoconstriction, increases coronary perfusion pressure, enhances the contractile state of the heart, stimulates spontaneous contractions, and increases the intensity of VF so increasing the likelihood of successful defibrillation.

The recommended IV/IO dose of adrenaline in children is 10 microgram kg^{-1}. The dose of adrenaline via the tracheal tube route is ten times the IV dose (100 microgram kg^{-1}). This route should be avoided if at all possible as evidence shows that there may be a paradoxical effect. Subsequent doses of adrenaline, if needed, should be given every 3-5 min. The use of a higher dose of adrenaline via the IV or IO route is not recommended routinely in children. High-dose adrenaline has not been shown to improve survival or neurological outcome after cardiopulmonary arrest.

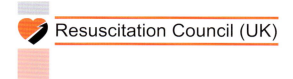

Amiodarone

Amoiodarone is a membrane-stabilising anti-arrhythmic drug that increases the duration of the action potential and refractory period in atrial and ventricular myocardium. Atrioventricular conduction is slowed, and a similar effect is seen with accessory pathways. Amiodarone has a mild negative inotropic action and causes peripheral vasodilation through non-competitive alpha-blocking effects. The hypotension that occurs with IV amiodarone is related to the rate of delivery and is due more to the solvent (Polysorbate 80), which causes histamine release, than the drug itself.

An initial IV dose of amiodarone 5 mg kg^{-1}, diluted in 5% dextrose, should be considered if VF or pulseless VT persists after a third shock. Amiodarone can cause thrombophlebitis when injected into a peripheral vein: use a central vein if a central venous catheter is in situ; if not, use a large peripheral vein and a generous flush of dextrose or saline.

Lidocaine

Until the publication of Guidelines 2000, lidocaine was the anti-arrhythmic drug of choice. Comparative studies with amiodarone have displaced it from this position and lidocaine is now recommended only for use when amiodarone is unavailable.

Atropine

When bradycardia is unresponsive to improved ventilation and circulatory support, atropine may be used. The dose of atropine is 20 microgram kg^{-1}, with a maximum dose of 600 microgram, and a minimum dose of 100 microgram to avoid a paradoxical effect at low doses.

Magnesium

This is a major intracellular cation and serves as a cofactor in a number of enzymatic reactions. Magnesium treatment is indicated in children with documented hypomagnesemia or with polymorphic VT ('torsade de pointes'), regardless of cause.

Give magnesium sulphate by intravascular infusion over several minutes, at a dose of 25 - 50 mg kg^{-1} (to a maximum of 2 g).

Calcium

Calcium plays a vital role in the cellular mechanisms underlying myocardial contraction, but there are very few data supporting any beneficial action of therapeutic calcium following most cases of cardiac arrest. High plasma concentrations achieved after injection may have detrimental effects on the ischaemic myocardium and may impair cerebral recovery. Thus, calcium is given during resuscitation only when specifically indicated, for example in

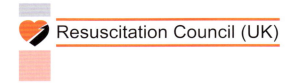

Resuscitation Council (UK)

hyperkalaemia, hypocalcaemia, and clinically severe overdose of calcium-channel-blocking drugs.

The dose of calcium chloride is 0.2 ml kg^{-1} of the 10% solution. Calcium can slow the heart rate and precipitate arrhythmias. In cardiac arrest, calcium may be given by rapid intravenous injection. In the presence of a spontaneous circulation it should be given slowly. Calcium solutions and sodium bicarbonate should not be administered simultaneously by the same route.

Sodium bicarbonate

Cardiac arrest results in combined respiratory and metabolic acidosis, caused by cessation of pulmonary gas exchange, and the development of anaerobic cellular metabolism respectively. The best treatment for acidaemia in cardiac arrest is a combination of chest compression and ventilation. Furthermore, giving bicarbonate causes generation of carbon dioxide which diffuses rapidly into the cells. This has the following effects:

- It exacerbates intracellular acidosis.
- It produces a negative inotropic effect on ischaemic myocardium.
- It presents a large, osmotically active, sodium load to an already compromised circulation and brain.
- It produces a shift to the left in the oxygen dissociation curve further inhibiting release of oxygen to the tissues.

The routine use of sodium bicarbonate in cardiac arrest is not recommended. It may be considered in prolonged arrest, and it has a specific role in hyperkalaemia and the arrhythmias associated with tricyclic antidepressant overdose. The dose is 1-2 ml kg^{-1} of the 8.4% solution given by the IV or IO routes.

Hypovolaemia

Hypovolaemia is a potentially reversible cause of cardiac arrest. If hypovolaemia is suspected, infuse intravenous or intraosseous fluids rapidly. In the initial stages of resuscitation there are no clear advantages in using colloid. Use isotonic saline solutions. Avoid dextrose-based solutions – these will be redistributed rapidly away from the intravascular space and will cause hyponatraemia and hyperglycaemia, which may worsen neurological outcome after cardiac arrest.

Therapeutic hypothermia

Mild hypothermia is thought to suppress many of the chemical reactions associated with reperfusion injury. Two randomised clinical trials showed improved outcome in adults remaining comatose after initial resuscitation from

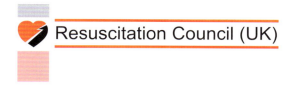

Resuscitation Council (UK)

out-of-hospital VF cardiac arrest. There are insufficient data for a firm recommendation for children.

Current guidance is that post-arrest infants and children with core temperatures less than 37.5°C should not be actively rewarmed, unless the core temperature is less than 33°C when they should be rewarmed to 34°C.

Hyperthermia has been shown to be correlated with a poorer outcome, so infants and children with core temperatures over 37.5°C should be actively cooled to a normal level. Shivering should be prevented by ensuring adequate sedation and giving neuromuscular blocking drugs.

Complications of mild therapeutic hypothermia include increased risk of infection, cardiovascular instability, coagulopathy, hyperglycaemia, and electrolyte abnormalities such as hypophosphataemia and hypomagnesaemia.

Parental Presence

Many parents would like to be present during a resuscitation attempt; they can see that everything possible is being done for their child. Reports show that being at the side of the child is comforting to the parents or carers, and helps them to gain a realistic view of attempted resuscitation and death. Families who have been present in the resuscitation room show less anxiety and depression several months after the death.

A dedicated staff member should be present with the parents at all times to explain the process in an empathetic and sympathetic manner. He or she can also ensure that the parents do not interfere with the resuscitation process or distract the medical and nursing staff. If the presence of the parents is impeding the progress of the resuscitation, they should be gently asked to leave. When appropriate, physical contact with the child should be allowed.

The team leader of the resuscitation, not the parents, will decide when to stop the resuscitation effort; this should be expressed with sensitivity and understanding. After the event, debriefing of the team should be conducted, to express any concerns and to allow the team to reflect on their clinical practice in a supportive environment.

References

1.   Efrati O, Ben-Abraham R, et al. Endobronchial adrenaline: should it be reconsidered? Dose response and haemodynamic effect in dogs. Resuscitation 2003; 59: 117-22.

2.   Newth C J, Rachman B, et al. The use of cuffed versus uncuffed endotracheal tubes in pediatric intensive care. J Pediatr 2004;144: 333-7.

3. Khine H H, Corddry D H, et al. Comparison of cuffed and uncuffed endotracheal tubes in young children during general anaesthesia. Anesthesiology 1997; 86: 627-631.

4. Van Alem A P, Chapman F W, et al. A prospective, randomised and blinded comparison of first shock success of monophasic and biphasic waveforms in out-of-hospital cardiac arrest. Resuscitation 2003; 58: 17-24.

5. Atkins D L, Jorgenson DB. Attenuated pediatric electrode pads for automated external defibrillators use in children. Resuscitation 2005; 66: 31-38.

6. Berg R A, Chapman FW, et al. Attenuated adult biphasic shocks compared with weight-based monophasic shocks in a swine model of prolonged pediatric ventricular fibrillation. Resuscitation 2004; 61: 189-197.

7. Clark C B, Zhang Y, et al. Pediatric transthoracic defibrillation: biphasic versus monophasic waveforms in an experimental model. Resuscitation 2001;51: 159-63.

8. Tang W, Weil M H, et al. Fixed-energy biphasic waveform defibrillation in a pediatric model of cardiac arrest and resuscitation. Crit Care Med 2002; 30: 2736-41.

9. Perondi M, Reis A, et al. A Comparison of High-Dose and Standard-Dose Epinephrine in Children with Cardiac Arrest. N Eng J Med 2004; 350: 1722-1730.

10. Patterson M D, Boenning DA, et al. The use of high-dose epinephrine for patients with out-of-hospital cardiopulmonary arrest refractory to prehospital interventions. Pediatr Emerg Care 2005; 21: 227-37.

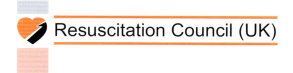

Newborn Life Support

Introduction

Passage through the birth canal is a hypoxic experience for the fetus, since significant respiratory exchange at the placenta is prevented for the 50-75 sec duration of the average contraction. Though most babies tolerate this well, the few that do not may require help to establish normal breathing at delivery. Newborn life support (NLS) is intended to provide this help and comprises the following elements:

- drying and covering the newborn baby to conserve heat;
- assessing the need for any intervention;
- opening the airway;
- lung aeration;
- rescue breathing;
- chest compression;
- administration of drugs (rarely).

Physiology

If subjected to continuing hypoxia in utero, the fetus will eventually lose consciousness and stop trying to 'breathe', as the neural centres controlling breathing cease to function due to lack of oxygen. The fetus then enters a period known as 'primary' apnoea.

Up to this point, the heart rate remains unchanged, but soon decreases to about half the normal rate as the myocardium reverts to anaerobic metabolism - a less fuel-efficient mechanism. The circulation to non-vital organs is reduced in an attempt to preserve perfusion of vital organs. The release of lactic acid, a by-product of anaerobic metabolism, causes deterioration of the biochemical milieu.

If the insult continues, shuddering, whole-body gasps at a rate of about 12 min^{-1} are initiated by primitive spinal centres. If these gasps fail to aerate the lungs they fade and the fetus enters a period known as 'secondary', or 'terminal', apnoea. Up until now, the circulation has been maintained but, as terminal apnoea progresses, the rapidly-deteriorating biochemical milieu begins to impair cardiac function. The heart eventually fails and, without effective intervention, the baby dies. The whole process probably takes almost twenty minutes in the term newborn human baby.

Thus, in the face of asphyxia, the baby can maintain an effective circulation throughout the period of primary apnoea, through the gasping phase, and even for a while after the onset of terminal apnoea. Thus, the most urgent requirement of any asphyxiated baby at birth is that the lungs be effectively aerated. Provided the baby's circulation is sufficiently intact, oxygenated blood will be conveyed from the aerated lungs to the heart. The heart rate will increase and the brain will

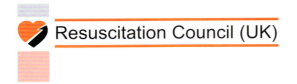

Newborn Life Support

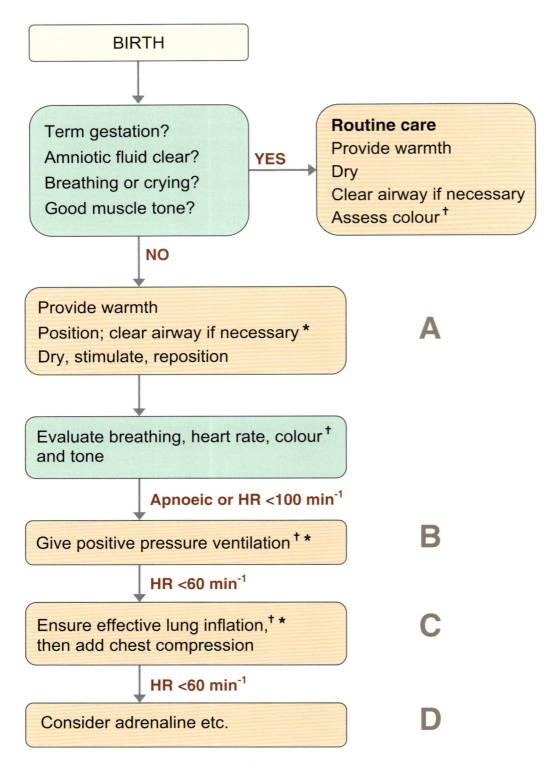

BIRTH

Term gestation?
Amniotic fluid clear?
Breathing or crying?
Good muscle tone?

YES →

Routine care
Provide warmth
Dry
Clear airway if necessary
Assess colour[†]

NO

Provide warmth
Position; clear airway if necessary[*]
Dry, stimulate, reposition

A

Evaluate breathing, heart rate, colour[†] and tone

Apnoeic or HR <100 min^{-1}

Give positive pressure ventilation[†][*]

B

HR <60 min^{-1}

Ensure effective lung inflation,[†][*] then add chest compression

C

HR <60 min^{-1}

Consider adrenaline etc.

D

[*] Tracheal intubation may be considered at several steps
[†] Consider supplemental oxygen at any stage if cyanosis persists

be perfused with oxygenated blood. Following this, the neural centres responsible for normal breathing will, in many instances, function once again and the baby will recover.

Merely aerating the lungs is sufficient in the vast majority of cases. However, though lung aeration is still vital, in a few cases cardiac function will have deteriorated to such an extent that the circulation is inadequate and cannot convey oxygenated blood from the aerated lungs to the heart. In this case, a brief period of chest compression may be needed. In a very few cases, lung aeration and chest compression will not be sufficient, and drugs may be required to restore the circulation. The outlook in this last group of infants is poor.

Guideline changes

The following are the main changes that have been made to the NLS guidelines:

- The use of food-grade plastic wrapping is recommended to maintain body temperature in significantly preterm babies.

- Attempts to aspirate meconium from the nose and mouth of the unborn baby, while the head is still on the perineum, is no longer recommended.

- Ventilatory resuscitation may be started with air. However, where possible, additional oxygen should be available if there is not a rapid improvement in the infant's condition.

- Adrenaline (epinephrine) should be given by the intravenous or intraosseous route, as standard doses are likely to be ineffective if given via a tracheal tube.

- If there are no signs of life after ten minutes of continuous and adequate resuscitation efforts, then discontinuation of resuscitation may be justified.

Sequence of actions

1 **Keep the baby warm and assess**

Babies are born small and wet. They get cold very easily, especially if they remain wet and in a draught.

- Whatever the problem, first make sure the cord is securely clamped and then dry the baby, remove the wet towels, and cover the baby with dry towels.

- For significantly preterm babies (30 weeks and below), there is now good evidence that placing the baby under a radiant heater and, without drying the baby beforehand, immediately covering the head and body, apart from the face, with food-grade plastic wrapping, is the most effective way of keeping these very small babies warm during resuscitation or stabilisation at birth.

- Drying the baby will provide significant stimulation and will allow time to assess colour, tone, breathing, and heart rate.

Reassess these observations regularly (particularly the heart rate) every 30 sec or so throughout the resuscitation process. The first sign of any improvement in the baby will be an increase in heart rate. Consider the need for help; if needed, ask for help immediately.

- A healthy baby will be born blue but will have good tone, will cry within a few seconds of delivery, will have a good heart rate (the heart rate of a healthy newborn baby is about 120-150 beats min^{-1}), and will rapidly become pink during the first 90 sec or so. A less healthy baby will be blue at birth, will have less good tone, may have a slow heart rate (less than 100 beats min^{-1}), and may not establish adequate breathing by 90-120 sec. An ill baby will be born pale and floppy, not breathing and with a slow or very slow heart rate.

- The heart rate of a baby is best judged by listening with a stethoscope. It can also be felt by gently palpating the umbilical cord but a slow rate at the cord is not always indicative of a truly slow heart rate - feeling for peripheral pulses is not helpful.

2   Airway

Before the baby can breathe effectively the airway must be open.

- The best way to achieve this is to place the baby on his back with the head in the neutral position, i.e. with the neck neither flexed nor extended. Most newborn babies will have a relatively prominent occiput, which will tend to flex the neck if the baby is placed on his back on a flat surface. This can be avoided by placing some support under the shoulders of the baby, but be careful not to overextend the neck.

- If the baby is very floppy it may also be necessary to apply chin lift or jaw thrust.

3   Breathing

- If the baby is not breathing adequately by about 90 seconds **give 5 inflation breaths.** Until now the baby's lungs will have been filled with fluid. Aeration of the lungs in these circumstances is likely to require sustained application of pressures of about 30 cm of water for 2-3 sec – these are 'inflation breaths'.

- If the heart rate was below 100 beats min^{-1} initially then it should rapidly increase as oxygenated blood reaches the heart. If the heart rate does increase then you can assume that you have successfully aerated the lungs. If the heart rate increases but the baby does not start breathing for himself, then continue to provide regular breaths at a rate of about 30-40 min^{-1} until the baby starts to breathe on his own.

- If the heart rate does not increase following inflation breaths, then either you have not aerated the lungs or the baby needs more than lung aeration alone. By far the most likely is that you have failed to aerate the lungs effectively. If the heart rate does not increase, and the chest does not passively move with each inflation breath, then you have not aerated the lungs.

- Consider:
    - Is the baby's head in the neutral position?
    - Do you need jaw thrust?
    - Do you need a longer inflation time?
    - Do you need a second person's help with the airway?
    - Is there an obstruction in the oropharynx (laryngoscope and suction)?
    - What about an oropharyngeal (Guedel) airway?

- Check that the baby's head and neck are in the neutral position, that your inflation breaths are at the correct pressure (30 cm of water) and applied for the correct time (2-3 sec inspiration), and that the chest moves with each breath. If the chest still does not move, ask for help in maintaining the airway and consider an obstruction in the oropharynx, which may be removable by suction under direct vision. An oropharyngeal (Guedel) airway may be helpful.

- If the heart rate remains slow (less than 60 min^{-1}) or absent following 5 inflation breaths, despite good passive chest movement in response to your inflation efforts, start chest compression.

4   Chest compression

Almost all babies needing help at birth will respond to successful lung inflation with an increase in heart rate followed quickly by normal breathing. However, in some cases chest compression is necessary.

- Chest compression should be started only when you are sure that the lungs have been aerated successfully.

- In babies, the most efficient method of delivering chest compression is to grip the chest in both hands in such a way that the two thumbs can press on the lower third of the sternum, just below an imaginary line joining the nipples, with the fingers over the spine at the back.

- Compress the chest quickly and firmly, reducing the antero-posterior diameter of the chest by about one third.

- **The ratio of compressions to inflations in newborn resuscitation is 3:1.**

- Chest compressions move oxygenated blood from the lungs back to the heart. Allow enough time during the relaxation phase of each compression cycle for the heart to refill with blood. Ensure that the chest is inflating with each breath.

In a very few babies inflation of the lungs and effective chest compression will not be sufficient to produce an effective circulation. In these circumstances drugs may be helpful.

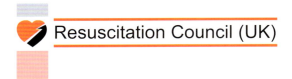
Resuscitation Council (UK)

5   Drugs

Drugs are needed only if there is no significant cardiac output despite effective lung inflation and chest compression.

- The drugs used are adrenaline (1:10,000), sodium bicarbonate (ideally 4.2%), and dextrose (10%). They are best delivered close to the heart, usually via an umbilical venous catheter.

- The recommended dose for adrenaline is 10 microgram kg^{-1} (0.1 ml kg^{-1} of 1:10,000 solution). If this is not effective a dose of up to 30 microgram kg^{-1} (0.3 ml kg^{-1} of 1:10,000 solution) may be tried.

- The dose for sodium bicarbonate is between 1 and 2 mmol of bicarbonate kg^{-1} (2 to 4 ml of 4.2% bicarbonate solution).

- The dose of dextrose recommended is 250 mg kg^{-1} (2.5 ml kg^{-1} of 10% dextrose).

- Very rarely, the heart rate cannot increase because the baby has lost significant blood volume. If this is the case, there is often a clear history of blood loss from the baby, but not always. Use of isotonic crystalloid rather than albumin is preferred for emergency volume replacement. A bolus of 10 ml kg^{-1} of 0.9% saline or similar given over 10 - 20 sec will often produce a rapid response and can be safely repeated if needed.

Explanatory Notes

Meconium

A large multicentre, randomised, controlled study[1] has shown that attempts to aspirate meconium from the nose and mouth of the unborn baby while the head is still on the perineum (so-called intrapartum suctioning) does not prevent meconium aspiration syndrome and this practice is no longer recommended. Another large multicentre, randomised, controlled study[2] has shown that attempts to remove meconium from the airways of vigorous babies after birth also fail to prevent this complication.

However, if babies are born through thick meconium and are unresponsive (or 'not vigorous') at birth, the oropharynx should be inspected and cleared of meconium. If intubation skills are available, the larynx and trachea should also be cleared. It is acknowledged that no proof of the efficacy of this practice exists.

Air or 100% oxygen

Concern about possible injurious effects of excess oxygen, particularly in preterm infants, and the apparent effectiveness of air in some limited, randomised, controlled, human studies of resuscitation at birth, has resulted in a minor change in the guidelines.

There is no evidence to suggest that any one concentration of oxygen is better than another when starting resuscitation. Some clinicians may wish to start with

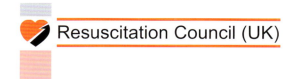
Resuscitation Council (UK)

air. However, where possible, it is recommended that additional oxygen should be available for use if there is not a rapid improvement in the infant's condition. Equally, hyperoxia should be avoided, especially in the preterm infant.

Route and dose of adrenaline

Adrenaline should be used in a concentration of 1:10,000 (100 microgram ml^{-1}). It is best given intravenously or by the intraosseous route. The standard recommended dose by these routes is 10 – 30 microgram kg^{-1} (0.1 – 0.3 ml kg^{-1} of 1:10,000). Do not use a higher dose by these routes as it is harmful.

Guidelines 2000 endorsed the use of adrenaline via the tracheal tube until an intravenous route had been established. Data now suggest that standard doses given via the tracheal tube are likely to be ineffective.

Induced hypothermia

Induced hypothermia may reduce the neurological damage associated with moderate post-asphyxial encephalopathy. However, as yet there are insufficient data to recommend routine use of modest systemic or selective cerebral hypothermia following resuscitation of infants with suspected asphyxia. Further randomised clinical trials are needed to determine which infants benefit most and which method of cooling is most effective.

References

1.   Vain NE, Szyld EG, Prudent LM, et al. Oropharyngeal and nasopharyngeal suctioning of meconium-stained neonates before delivery of their shoulders: multicentre, randomised controlled trial. Lancet 2004: 364; 597-602.

2.   Wiswell TE, Gannon CM, Jacob J, et al. Delivery room management of the apparently vigorous meconium-stained neonate: results of the multicenter international collaborative trial. Pediatr 2000; 105: 1-7.

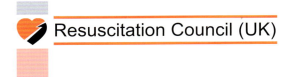

Resuscitation Council (UK)